BASIC COMMUNITY AND HOME CARE NURSING

Mary K. Ringsven, R.N.C., B.A.
Barbara M. Jorenby, R.N., B.S.N.

DELMAR PUBLISHERS INC.®

perform any independent analysis in connection with any of the product information contained herein. Publisher does not assume, and expressly disclaims, any obligation to obtain and include information other than that provided to it by the manufacturer.

The reader is expressly warned to consider and adopt all safety precautions that might be indicated by the activities described herein and to avoid all potential hazards. By following the instructions contained herein, the reader willingly assumes all risks in connection with such instructions.

The publisher makes no representations or warranties of any kind, including but not limited to, the warranties of fitness for particular purpose or merchantability, nor are any such representations implied with respect to the material set forth herein, and the publisher takes no responsibility with respect to such material. The publisher shall not be liable for any special, consequential or exemplary damages resulting, in whole or in part, from the readers' use of, or reliance upon, this material.

Photography by David Thelen
TruColor Studio, Farmington, MN

Delmar Staff
   Administrative Editor: Leslie Boyer
   Managing Editor: Barbara Christie
   Production Editor: Ruth East
   Design Coordinator: Susan Mathews
   Publications Coordinator: Karen Seebald

For information, address Delmar Publishers Inc.
2 Computer Drive West, Box 15-015
Albany, New York 12212

COPYRIGHT © 1988
BY DELMAR PUBLISHERS INC.

All rights reserved. No part of this work covered by the copyright hereon may be reproduced or used in any form or by any means—graphic, electronic, or mechanical, including photocopying, recording, taping, or information storage and retrieval systems—without written permission of the publisher.

Printed in the United States of America
Published simultaneously in Canada
by Nelson Canada,
a division of International Thomson Limited

10 9 8 7 6 5 4 3 2

Library of Congress Cataloging in Publication Data

Ringsven, Mary K., 1940–
  Basic community and home care nursing.

  Bibliography: p.
  Includes index.
  1. Community health nursing—United States. 2. Home nursing—United States. 3. Community health nursing—Vocational guidance. 4. Home nursing—Vocational guidance. I. Jorenby, Barbara M. II. Title. [DNLM: 1. Community Health Nursing. 2. Home Care Services. WY 106 R582b]
RT98.R56   1988   610.73′43   87-8995
ISBN 0-8273-2969-5 (soft)
ISBN 0-8273-2970-9 (instructor's guide)

CONTENTS

Preface vii

SECTION ONE: THE HEALTH CARE DELIVERY SYSTEM

UNIT 1   NURSING IN THE TWENTY-FIRST
CENTURY 3
Anticipated changes in health care
The changing roles of caregivers
The changes in patient care

UNIT 2   HEALTH CARE DELIVERY
SYSTEM 12
Defining the health care delivery system
History of the system
Levels of intervention
Public policy and the health care system

UNIT 3   PAYING FOR HEALTH CARE 35
Payment alternatives
Cost containment
Effects of cost containment

UNIT 4   EXPANDED SETTINGS FOR HEALTH CARE
DELIVERY 50
Changing care in traditional settings
New settings for acute care
New settings for long term care
Expanded use of home health care
Factors influencing the choice of care setting

UNIT 5   HOME HEALTH CARE: A RETURNING
ALTERNATIVE 64
Historical review
Home health care today

Types of home health care programs
How a home health care agency works

SECTION TWO: COMMUNITIES' RESPONSIBILITY FOR HEALTH CARE

UNIT 6   COMMUNITIES AND THEIR HEALTH 78
Defining communities
Looking at world-wide health concerns
Looking at U.S. health concerns
Additional communities identified
Community involvement in health concerns
Identifying and resolving community health risks
Nurses in the community

UNIT 7   THE TEAM CONCEPT OF COMMUNITY AND HOME CARE 94
Defining the community health care team
Developing a comprehensive health care team
Implementing successful teamwork
Reaching the goal of the comprehensive health care team
Identifying the nurse's role

UNIT 8   COMMUNITY AND HOME CARE TEAM MEMBERS 107
Identifying team members and roles in home health care
Cultural influences on health care
Family influences on health care

SECTION THREE: NURSES AND THEIR PATIENTS IN THE COMMUNITY

UNIT 9   ADAPTING BASIC NURSING CONCEPTS TO EXPANDED SETTINGS 136
Using the nursing process
Considering the patient's basic needs
Identifying changes through the life span
Additional concepts for adaptation

UNIT 10 APPLYING BASIC CONCEPTS TO PRACTICE IN EXPANDED SETTINGS 163
Working in a clinic or office setting
Working in an ambulatory surgery center
Working in a home health care setting

CONTENTS

          Working in day care for the elderly or handicapped
          Working in respite care
          Working in a hospice

UNIT 11 NURSE'S RESPONSIBILITIES TO SELF AND CAREER 185
          Understanding yourself
          Job seeking
          Issues to consider

UNIT 12 NURSES' INFLUENCING FUTURE HEALTH CARE 202
          Health promotion
          Issues of quality care and access
          Political involvement

APPENDIX A   NURSING DIAGNOSES 217
APPENDIX B   HOME HEALTH CARE: SAMPLE ASSESSMENT AND CARE PLAN 221
GLOSSARY 227
BIBLIOGRAPHY 233
INDEX 239

PREFACE

The concept for writing this book grew out of projects and curriculum development which have occupied us for some time. In 1984 one of the authors received project funding to develop curriculum in Community and Home Care Nursing for a practical nursing program. While researching related literature, she discovered that texts for community health nursing are written primarily for public health nurses and social workers. Yet it was learned that many agencies employ nurse generalists in home health care. And it is obvious that many nurses are employed in offices and clinics, although most curricula do not significantly address that area. The other author was involved in a "Project '88," which explored possible changes needed in practical nursing education to better prepare graduates. A survey of Minnesota hospital and nursing home directors indicated that nurses need better preparation in communication skills and management techniques. It also indicated that no one wants to predict the future of nursing education!

We realize that nursing education must change as health care changes. Although we are presently involved in one level of education, we appreciate the other levels. The direct-care nurse we envision will be a new type, a combination of the best of present types. It is for this nurse that this book is intended.

Nursing education should prepare graduates for their future roles as well as present situations. We believe in the need for quality caregivers, educated to make observations and perform technical skills as well as to give care and follow the plans established by professionals. We also believe that home health care agencies will come to view this nurse as cost-effective.

Basic Community and Home Care Nursing does not teach basic caregiving skills. Giving a bath or medication in the home is not much different from giving them in a hospital. Explaining formula preparation to a new mother does not change when the nurse works in a clinic. This text encourages nurses to view health care in a wider scope. We look briefly at the history of the system and explore the present reimbursement problems. We discuss community in the broadest sense and explore the expanded settings of health care delivery. We include some examples of how nurses can practice in some of these new settings.

Employers indicate that nurses newly entering home health care need strengthening of these skills: listening and in-depth communication, observation of family interaction, identification of chemical dependency and other abuses, and independent problem solving. We have addressed all these areas, realizing that each could be an entire course of its own!

Basic Community and Home Care Nursing can be used near the end of a one- or two-year nursing program. Ideally, a practicum experience in community and/or home health care should be correlated with the text. *Basic Community and Home Care Nursing* may also be useful to nurses who are entering community or home health care after practicing in other areas. We have made every attempt to present accurate information relative to government regulations and standards of practice at the time of publication.

ACKNOWLEDGMENTS

We are grateful to the many people who helped us make this book a reality: Mary Jane Swinton, who encouraged the initial curriculum projects. Penny Siven, who insisted we could and should write. Other colleagues who offered moral support and encouragement: Sandra Robertson, Rae Brooks, Lib McDonough, Karen Blackstad, and Sandra Thomsen.

Of course, our families contributed much to our efforts: Ron, Sharon, and Brian Ringsven; Bob, Charles, and Curt Jorenby. They helped us learn word processing and relieved us of many homemaking tasks during this time.

We also want to thank our editor, Leslie Boyer, for her enthusiastic support. We want to thank Delmar reviewers for their comments, which helped us shape the final manuscript. In addition, thanks are due to many health care facilities and professionals for their numerous contributions to this project.

Our thanks to Regina Medical Complex, including Quality Home Care in Hastings, MN, for permitting us to photograph in their extended care areas; and staff members Mary Hale, RN, Dee Churchill, PHN, Barbara E. Kendall, RN, and Carrie Anibas. Thanks also to the River Valley Clinic, Hastings, MN, and staff, Leslie Atwood, MD, William Spinelli, MD, Thomas Schwinghamer, MD, Kris Swanson, RN, Suzanne Werner, LPN, and Debbie and Danita Eggers.

We also want to thank Twyla Geiken, the TRAC bus driver, and the Hastings senior citizen congregate dining group. Thanks to the students

PREFACE

and graduates of the practical nursing program and the supportive friends who agreed to be in photographs: Steve Langenfeld, LPN, Coralee Nelson, LPN, Nancy Waller, LPN, Maxine Logan, Perry H. Hultin, Jennifer Robinson-West, Jessie Glosson, Randy Sticha, Vivian Enander, Sam and Donna Sorenson, the Rev. David W. Rossow, and James and Bette Clement, Sara and Matthew.

Special thanks go to Leon and Barbara Budahl for allowing us to bring a photographer into their home. It was important to us to show readers the "real" situation and the home care team. This included Maureen Budahl, Peter and Elizabeth, and Patricia Steiger, RN.

Mary K. Ringsven
Barbara M. Jorenby

SECTION ONE

THE HEALTH CARE DELIVERY SYSTEM

Unit 1 Nursing in the Twenty-first Century
Unit 2 The Health Care Delivery System
Unit 3 Paying for Health Care
Unit 4 Expanded Settings for Health Care Delivery
Unit 5 Home Health Care: A Returning Alternative

Nurses are expanding their horizons in the type of patient care practiced, where the care is given, and in the authority they have over the care given. Nursing is gaining a still stronger voice in planning patient care. Nurses are evolving into more active health team members, figure 1–1.

The current health care delivery system expects nurses to become more involved in the business aspect of the system. They are expected to be efficient and economical and be aware of time and costs. Still, quality care remains the top priority.

Looking at the past helps put the future into perspective. The road to practice in tomorrow's expanded settings will be clearer after you have viewed the progression of the health care delivery system.

Section One sets the stage. The units present a brief history of health care in the United States: where people were helped, who assisted them, and how the costs were met. The section concludes with recent changes in health care delivery in expanded settings and the return to home health care.

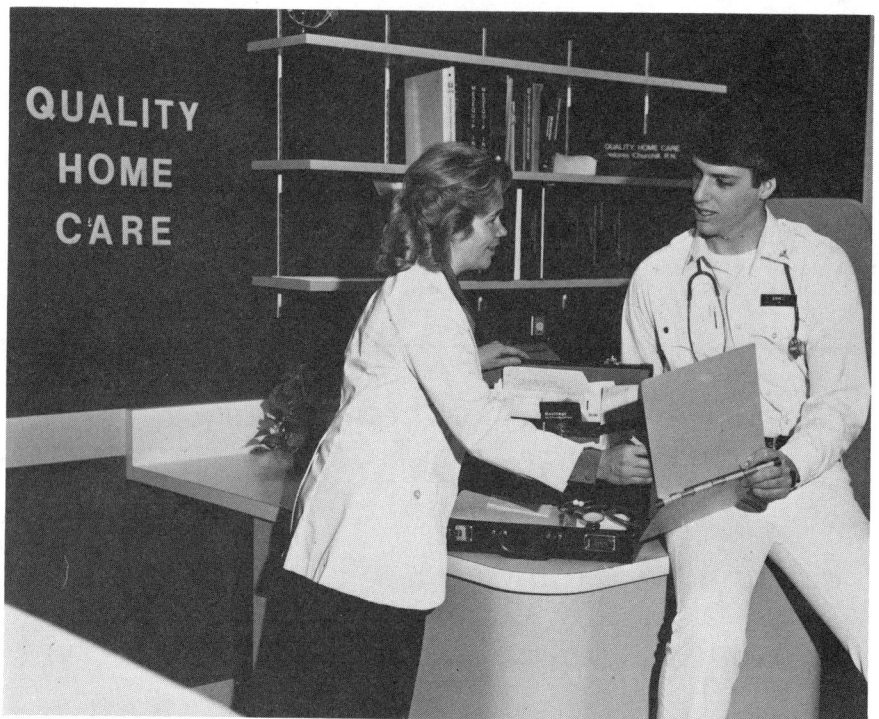

Figure 1–1 Home health care will expand in the 21th century.

1

Nursing in the Twenty-First Century

OBJECTIVES:

After completing this unit, you will be able to:

- Identify four changes in the future of health care.
- Identify three changes in the roles of nurses.
- Explain at least two ways in which patient care will change.
- Define and give one example of the nurse generalist.
- Define the term *case coordinator*.

Welcome to the 21st century! Well, almost. The 21st century is not far away. Futurists predict many changes in all aspects of daily life. Health care is not exempt from changes, and nursing must prepare now to meet those changes. This unit will look at some projected changes in how health care is provided, in the roles of health care workers, and in patient care, Figure 1–1.

ANTICIPATED CHANGES IN HEALTH CARE

One change already occurring is that individuals are much more involved in taking care of their health. Americans have always wanted to be in control of their own lives, and this desire will not diminish in the future. As people become better educated in healthy lifestyles, more of them work at staying fit and controlling excess weight. More persons will grow up understanding the importance of nutrition, exercise, and stress in their lives. Many will also become more aware of the cost of being ill. More employers will reward their workers for staying healthy instead of paying for absenteeism due to sickness.

Another change foreseen is that health care will become more *decentralized*. Instead of only large hospitals serving a geographical area, there will also be many smaller facilities. More *entrepreneurs* will offer services in new ways. Entrepreneurs are persons who organize and manage a new business venture which may have a risk involved. Competition among services is already becoming commonplace. Figure 1-2 is an example of recent health care advertising. The marketing of health care services continues to be an expanding area.

The federal government will become more involved in health care. Whether regulation will improve health care or not is a matter of concern. Who should decide the right kind of health care for America?

Alternate types of facilities will become even more common. Large clinics will provide many of the services formerly found only in hospitals. The location of emergency centers near busy freeways, and the helicopter transfer of patients will be commonplace. Already there are many ambulatory surgery centers where patients enter in the morning, have surgery, recover, and go home the same day. At times these are part of hospitals, but not always. Walk-in doctors' offices will gain in popularity.

Patients may be able to call their doctors on computers, answer questions and describe symptoms, and the doctor will send a prescription out to them. If more information is needed, the videophone can help the doctor examine the patient more thoroughly; for example, "Put the camera closer to that sore toe, please." A computer view of future health care is shown in figure 1-3.

Hospitals currently used for acute care will be used only for the most critically ill patients; specialists will manage patient care with even more machinery than is used now. Meals will be delivered by robots, and medications by conveyor belts. The immune system will be understood and managed, so that transplants of major organs will be easier. More artificial organs will be developed. A balance between advancing technology and increasing costs will be needed. Patients will be discharged from these hospitals as soon as they are stable. Some may go to convalescent facilities; some will be sent home.

Long term care will also be different. The nursing home industry that developed in the '60s and '70s segregated the elderly from the rest of the population, sometimes without regard for their degree of health. Gerontological knowledge has demonstrated that many elderly can be better cared for in alternate settings such as group homes. Future long term care facilities for the elderly will focus on the oldest segment, those over 85, who tend to be the most dependent.

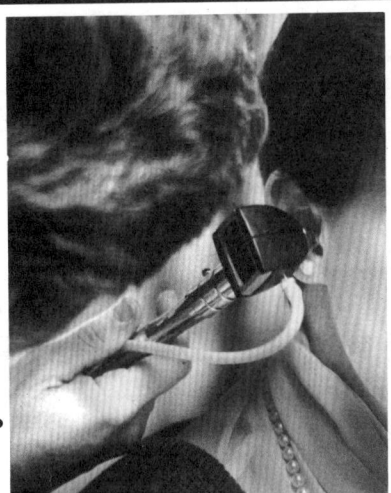

Figure 1–2 Example of recent health care advertising (Courtesy of Regina Medical Complex, Hastings, Minnesota)

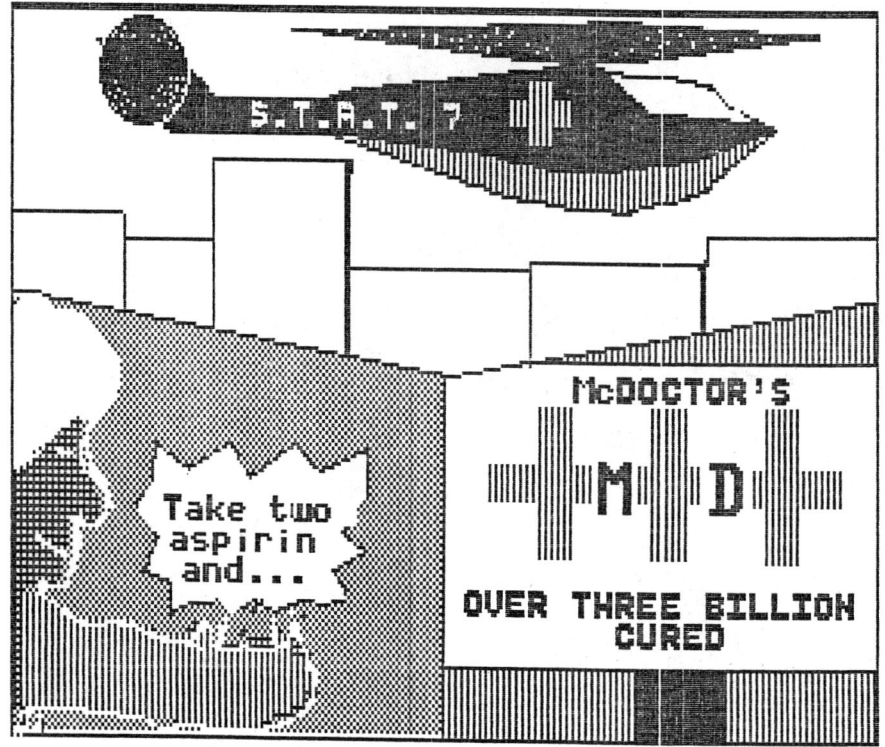

Figure 1–3 A computer view of future health care (Coutesy of Curt Jorenby)

Some long term care facilities now care for people who have been discharged from hospitals but continue to need skilled nursing care. This trend will increase in the future. There will also be more community residences for other groups such as the mentally handicapped, the physically disabled, and the mentally ill.

Other changes which can be predicted include the extension of office and clinic hours to 24 hours a day, seven days a week. Caregivers may become more mobile, traveling to patients in rural areas. Home health care will continue to increase and will become regulated by state or federal government. Generally, illness will be treated at home. Even complex therapies may be treated at home with the right kind of management.

Payment methods will change as well. Will employers offer birth-to-death wellness programs as a part of health coverage? Should employers provide coverage for employees and dependents? Who should pay for long term care? Will our society have to develop new ways to pay for care of the unemployed, poor, or indigent? Will there be a National Health Care Policy?

UNIT 1/NURSING IN THE TWENTY-FIRST CENTURY

The health care industry will continue to grow as one of the largest industries in the country. As the number of people over 70 increases, more specialists in geriatrics will be needed. Figure 1–4 shows predicted changes in population age groups. The industry will need many kinds of workers at all levels of care. Communities with an active health care industry will be economically sound.

KEY CONCEPT: CHANGES IN HEALTH CARE

- More individual responsibility
- Greater decentralization
- Entrepreneurs, newer ways of giving care
- Increased home health care
- More government regulations
- Continued growth of health care industry

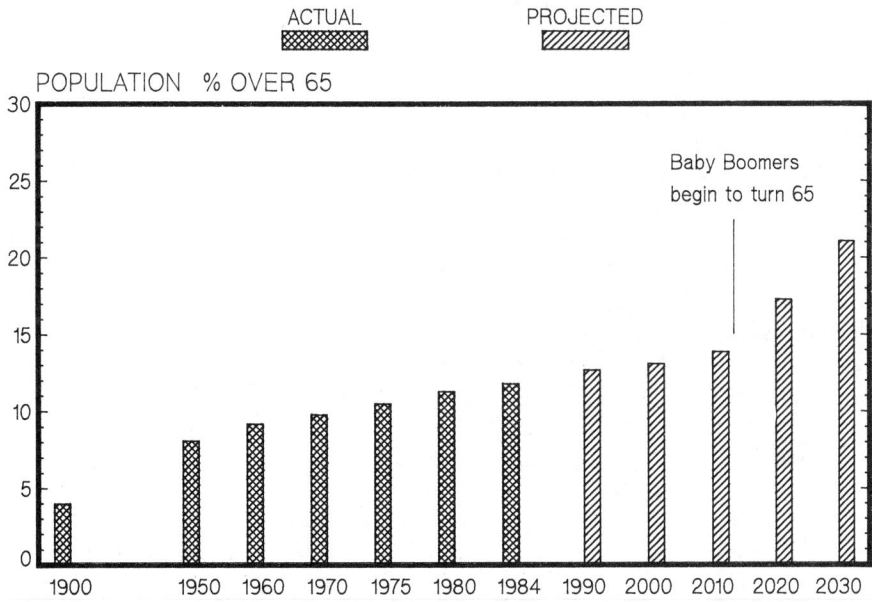

Figure 1–4 Predicting population changes (Data Source: U.S. Department of Commerce, Bureau of the Census)

THE CHANGING ROLES OF CAREGIVERS

Nurses and other caregivers will also find their roles changing. Acute care hospitals will bill separately for nursing care, which means every level of nursing will become precisely accountable for the care that is given.

Nurse generalists will be in demand. A *generalist* is someone who has a good understanding of many areas, but has not specialized in one area. A nurse generalist will have a basic nursing education, know about many common health problems and therapies, and understand human behavior. Most new graduates are beginning generalists. Nurses who have worked in traditional medical–surgical settings with a variety of patients also can be called generalists.

Nurse generalists will continue to be the support staff of hospitals, long term care facilities, and many expanding settings of health care delivery. As technology increases, they will need to become more skilled with computerized equipment. However, patients will always need personalized care given by another person.

Nurses with special clinical education will continue to be in demand for Intensive Care Units and other specialties. Nurses with advanced degrees who are independent nurse practitioners may have staff privileges in hospitals and long term care facilities. They will shift from being primary caregivers to roles of health educators and case coordinators. Some will be in practice as partners with physicians.

Physicians of the future will also find their roles changing. Many will be salaried employees of Health Maintenance Organizations. Others will be employed by large corporations to manage wellness programs. The increasing concern for wellness will lead many physicians into public teaching.

Doctors will be part of the total team for health care, but they will not necessarily be the leader. Other health care professionals will also develop and move into new roles in the future. Physical therapists will find their roles growing, especially in helping more older people maintain a level of wellness while coping with chronic problems. Many therapists will also work in schools to help children with physical disabilities. Pharmacists may well distribute medications directly to homes on a regular route. As an example, an orthodontist in northern Wisconsin has had a motor home equipped to serve as his office. He regularly travels to numerous small communities to see his patients.

As every professional role grows and changes, support workers will be needed to assist them. Some of these positions are just beginning to evolve.

> ### KEY CONCEPT: CHANGES IN ROLES
>
> - Nurse generalists considered important
> - Many more independent nurses
> - Physicians viewed as team members
> - Roles expanded in new ways
> - Many support workers needed

THE CHANGES IN PATIENT CARE

Increasing technology will require greater knowledge by all health care workers. As more equipment becomes computerized, everyone who is working with the affected patient needs to be knowledgeable about the machinery and comfortable with its operation. Patients don't need helpers who are afraid of their equipment! Some people already live at home with kangaroo pumps for gastrostomy feedings. Portable oxygen units can be seen in use in churches and shopping centers. Even motorized wheelchairs are becoming a part of everyday life.

Patients will also need to learn more about their own health care. In many situations, patients will be the decision makers about the treatment to be done. They need to understand their medications and side effects. If they leave the hospital earlier after surgery, they must know the signs of post-operative complications that might occur. Compliance with their own health care regimen requires that patients understand the outcomes of continuing or not continuing treatment.

Advances in research and development will lead to new and improved treatments. Medications will be targeted to go directly to the diseased organ. Genetic research will help make many birth defects past history. Diagnoses will be made more quickly, and the specific treatment will be started immediately. Computers will be available for every home and office, and most people will be able to use them knowledgeably. Communication between health care experts will be immediate.

All of this technology may be reassuring for the patient who is ill or it may be frightening. Health care may become "high-tech," but people will always need "high-touch," especially when ill. Machinery can give us reams of data, but it doesn't furnish reassuring smiles or give a backrub! We know today that the patient's emotional state is vital in the recovery and maintenance of health. It is very unlikely that that will ever change.

In future acute care settings, it will be the nurse generalist who will be the crucial link between the patient and the machinery. It is necessary to know about the machinery, but the patient must remain more important.

In many of the future expanded settings for health care, the patient will become his or her own *case coordinator*. A case coordinator is the person who organizes home health care according to the needs of the patient. Numerous choices for health care will be available. To learn about possible choices, the patient will often turn to the most accessible caregiver, which may be you!

Families will also need knowledge about caring for each other. Many more people will receive health care in their homes. The nurse will have an important role in helping families learn. It will be necessary to know about diverse cultural and ethnic groups in the United States. Some members of these groups may not adopt the traditional methods for health care, yet their needs must be met.

KEY CONCEPT: CHANGES IN CARE

- Increased knowledge needed by all
- Patients manage their own care
- Increased technology
- Rapid diagnosis
- Growing home health care

SUMMARY

The future of health care is closely bound with the future of the nation and of society as a whole. While the federal government looks at additional regulations, patients are taking over their own care and becoming responsible for their own health. As technology increases, the roles of doctors, nurses, other health care workers, patients, and families will change. This will require greater knowledge by everyone involved. More health care will be given in the home. There will also continue to be a great need for the human touch provided by competent nurses.

FOR DISCUSSION

- What are some ways in which people in your community can become better educated about their responsibility for their own health?
- What resources exist in your community to learn more about advancing technology?
- Explain what is meant by the term *"nurse generalist."* Do you consider yourself a generalist?
- Imagine you are employed in a hospital in the year 2010. What kinds of responsibilities will you have? What kinds of problems will patients have?

QUESTIONS FOR REVIEW

1. What are four changes predicted for health care in the future?
2. List three changes predicted in the roles of nurses.
3. Give two examples of future changes in patient care.
4. Define *nurse generalist* and *case coordinator*.

2

Health Care Delivery System

OBJECTIVES:

After completing this unit, you will be able to:

- Define the health care delivery system.
- Discuss how historical eras affected health care.
- Identify two health crises in the United States.
- Explain the four levels of health care intervention.
- Identify nursing's role in each level of intervention.
- Discuss how the nation's political structure affects health care delivery.

Nurses at all levels of practice need to have a basic understanding of the health care delivery system in the United States in order to be more active participants. The system has four components: (1) the goods and services themselves, (2) the delivery of those goods and services, (3) the use of the goods and services, and (4) the funding of the system.

The present decentralized system with its numerous care settings makes nurses wonder where they will be practicing and what they will be doing. This unit will explain where nursing has historically fit into the overall system. Why do problems occur? Why are changes needed? Why are changes difficult to make?

Four levels of health care intervention will then be discussed, including how nurses are involved at each level. Public policy and its effects on the health care delivery system is also included.

DEFINING THE HEALTH CARE DELIVERY SYSTEM

The *health care delivery system* refers to the entire health care industry that exists to meet all the health needs of the nation. The first of the four-part system is the goods and services needed for health care. This means companies that manufacture equipment and supplies—from thermometers to surgical instruments, from chart forms to pill bottles. It also means pharmaceutical companies and publishers of health education materials. It includes the services of health care workers and the schools and educators who taught them.

The next part of the system applies to the delivery of goods and services to the people who need them. This includes traditional institutions such as hospitals, nursing homes, clinics, and agencies that provide health care at home. There are also new ways being developed to deliver health care goods and services.

The third part of the system applies to the people who need the health care goods and services. This includes the methods of distribution, knowledge of who are receiving services, and how the services are given. A delivery method may be designed for the distribution of goods, but if the people who need the service don't use it, they won't benefit from it. Whether or not people use the institutions for health care is one measure of the effectiveness of the system as a whole.

The last part of the system applies to the financing of these goods and services. Sometimes individuals pay for their own care. Many times employers and health insurance companies help pay for health care. State and federal governments are also involved in payment arrangements. Indirectly, paying for health care means paying for thermometers and chart forms and many other things, whether the care is delivered in traditional settings or in a new way.

KEY CONCEPT: DEFINITION

- Part 1: Goods and Services
- Part 2: Delivery of goods and services
- Part 3: Use of goods and services
- Part 4: Payment for goods and services

HISTORY OF THE SYSTEM

Overview

Health care in the United States was modeled after health care as it was practiced in Europe. Immigrant groups brought along their cultural beliefs and practices about health care and medicine. Physicians were in charge of all health education but folk medicine was widely accepted and practiced.

As the nation grew, new approaches to health care were developed. Hospitals became the centers for care of the sick; health resources were used more liberally. In Europe, socialized medicine provided for the care of most ill people. In the United States, those who could afford care received it. Those who could not afford it sometimes had to do without.

The rapid growth of technology in all areas also had its effect on health care practices. Specialization grew, requiring more and more money. Not only did physicians specialize in general or internal medicine, but specialties became divided even further. Plastic surgery, for example, was divided into head, neck, nose, or hand specialties!

Organization of Health Services

America's founding fathers established our government based upon *Federalism*—local government was preferred over a national system. This also applied to health care delivery; each community or state was supposed to take care of its citizens. Being self-sufficient was the ideal.

However, original welfare laws grew out of the tradition of the English Poor Laws. People who, through some misfortune, were not able to provide for their own needs, would be cared for by the local government.

The effects of this early philosophy on today's health care delivery are easily illustrated. We are one of the few industrialized nations in the world that do not have a national health policy for all of its citizens. State laws for the care of the poor are not uniform; this helps explain the unequal quality of care in various geographical areas.

The Nineteenth Century

Society in the early nineteenth century (1800–1850) centered around the family. Illnesses were treated at home, often with home remedies. When the family could not care for the sick person themselves, they usually had a neighbor who was qualified because of previous experiences. Nursing was considered an extension of the mother's duties of nurturing and caregiving.

Some Catholic Sisterhoods gave novices a few months of training in home nursing. Figure 2–1A and 2–1B depict changes in nursing education.

"Poor Houses" were established near larger communities to care for the needy and the indigent. Sometimes these were operated by churches or other charitable organizations. People in need were given food and whatever care was necessary and available.

During the latter part of the nineteenth century (1850–1900), health care for the most part continued to be given in the home. Physicians who had attended an approved medical college were considered true professionals. In 1800 there were four medical schools in the U.S.; in 1850 there were forty-two. Licensure of physicians became accepted by the end of the century.

Hospitals also grew in number. Some were established by doctors, some were built by communities, and some were extensions of medical schools. Still, people avoided hospitals whenever possible. Until Ignaz Filipp Semmelweis and Joseph Lister proved their "germ" theories, hospitals were not very healthy places.

Nursing gradually came into its own in this country after Florence Nightingale became well known in England. The Civil War demonstrated the need for large numbers of nurses. Much of battlefield nursing was done by soldiers with minor wounds. Volunteer nurses helped during the War; these women were not trained as nurses, however. After the Civil War, the American Hospital Association said that all large hospitals should train their own nurses. Educated women who were wealthy and single were considered good potential nurses.

The first school for practical nursing was established in 1892 in New York; it was a three-month program. Graduates gave basic nursing care to people in their homes and helped with hygiene and nutrition. Figure 2–2 on page 18 illustrates early nursing care in a home.

Hospital training programs ranged from one to two years in length. Graduates of the early hospital training schools became head nurses and instructors. Students provided most of the staffing. In 1893 there were 47 hospital schools of nursing in the country. Figure 2–3 on page 19 illustrates the responsibilities of hospital nurses a century ago.

The Twentieth Century

Care of people with illnesses began moving more into hospitals after the turn of the century. Medicine continued to be an honored profession. A major reason why a boy might finish high school and go to college was to practice medicine.

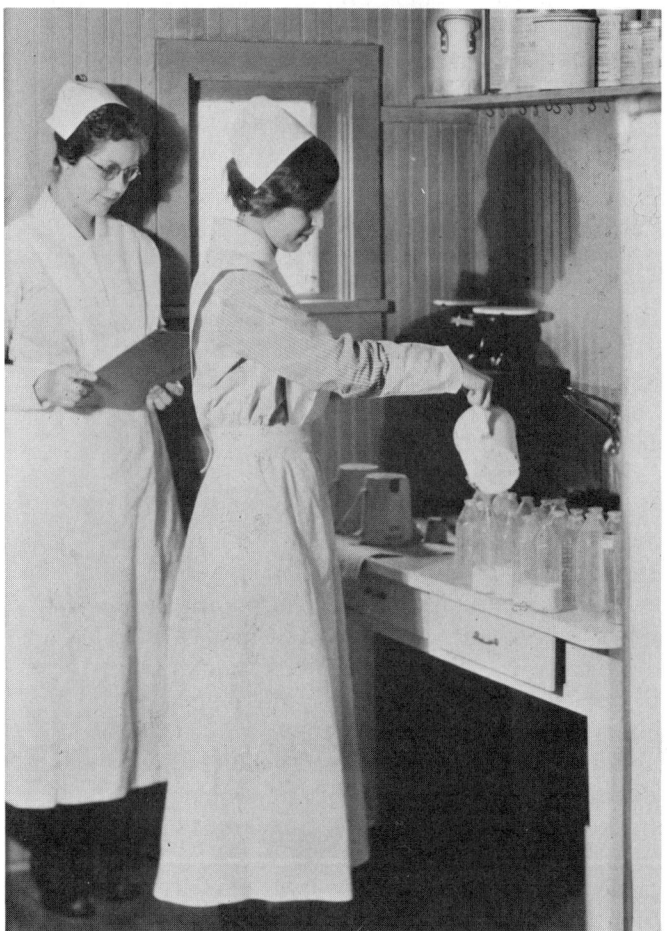

Figure 2–1a Nursing education then (Courtesy of the Minnesota Historical Society)

The Early Years (1900–1940) Early feminists and visionary nursing leaders tried to improve nurses' education and image by moving training programs into college settings. One of the first college nursing programs was at the University of Minnesota, where student nurses studied liberal arts and worked 56 hours a week in the hospital as well! Although some other colleges and universities added nursing programs, progress was slow.

In 1903, nursing practice was recognized as worthy of legislative control and the first permissive laws were passed. *Permissive laws* gave require-

UNIT 2/HEALTH CARE DELIVERY SYSTEM

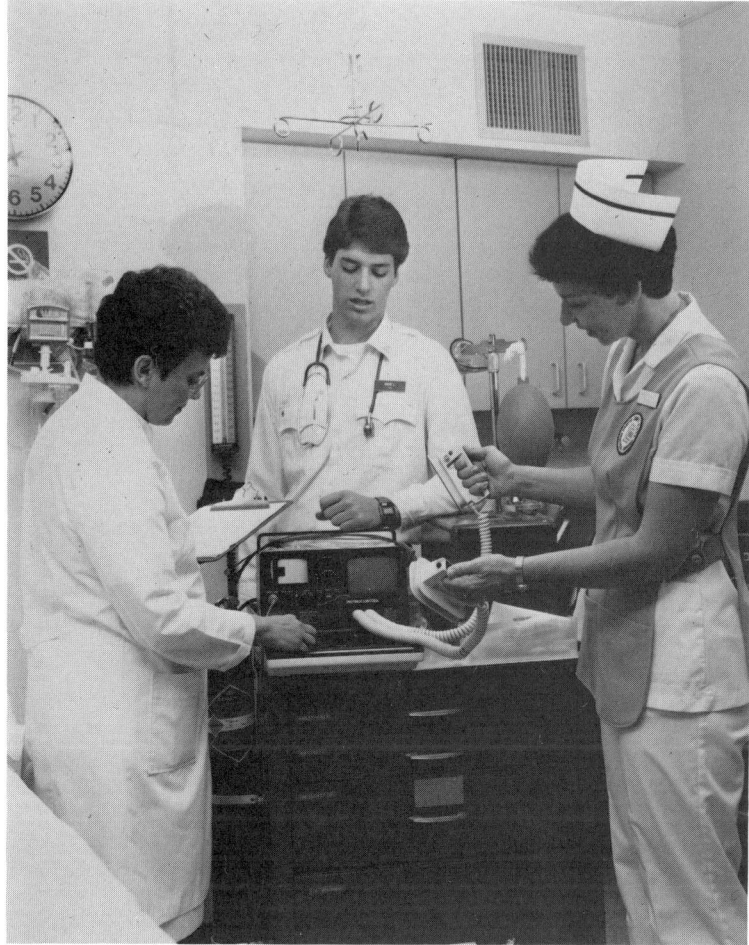

Figure 2–1b Nursing education now

ments for those nurses who wanted to have licenses, but did not restrict nursing practice to licensed persons. In 1914 Mississippi was the first state to enact a law controlling practical nursing education. In 1919 the first practical nurse program in a high school was started at the Minneapolis Girls Vocational High School.

World War I created a huge demand for more nurses, so more hospitals began training programs. The criteria were less strict to encourage more students. There was not much uniformity of these programs, so in 1923

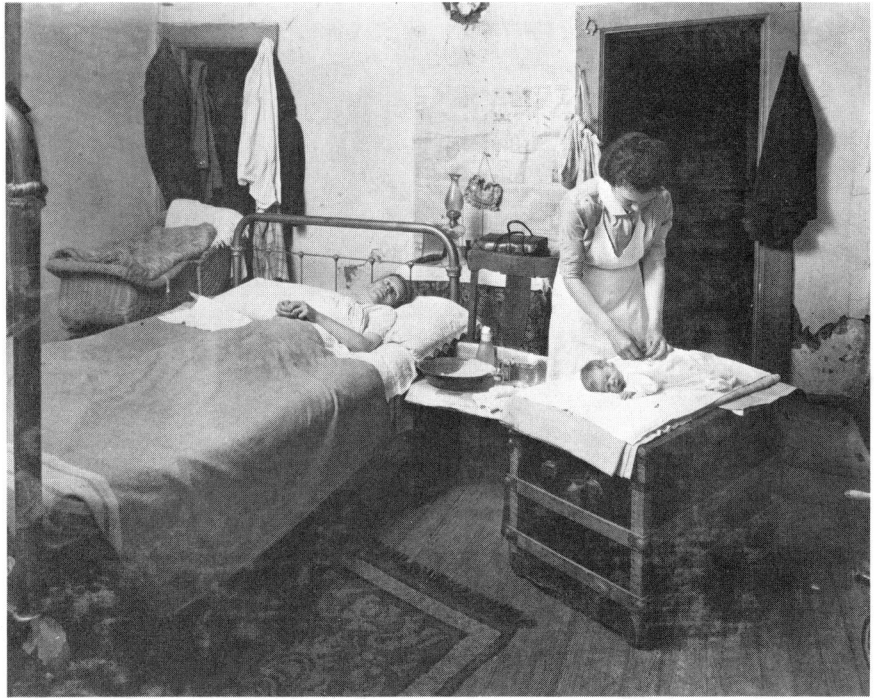

Figure 2–2 Early home care nursing (Courtesy of the Minnesota Historical Society)

leading nurse educators agreed on a 28-month program that would include public health training. Students lived in nurses' residences and could not marry while in training. Figure 2–4 identifies some leaders in American nursing.

The economic Depression left its effects on the social scene, with the government initiating many programs to help with recovery. The Social Security Act of 1935 included funding for three particular health programs: maternal and child health, medical care for crippled children, and child welfare programs. These programs were administered through the states. Much of the focus was on improving the health of mothers and children, particularly in rural areas, which were viewed as underserved.

The Middle Years (1940–1960) World War II contributed to medical practices in many ways. As the weapons became more sophisticated, battle wounds became more severe. The birth of antibiotics contributed to greater

In addition to caring for your 50 patients, each nurse will follow these regulations:

- Daily sweep and mop the floor of your ward, dust the patient furniture and window sills.
- Maintain an even temperature in your ward by bringing in a scuttle of coal for the day's business.
- Light is important to observe the patient's condition; therefore, each day fill kerosene lamps, clean chimneys, and trim wicks. Wash the windows once a week.
- The nurses' notes are important in aiding the physician's work. Make your pens carefully; you may whittle the nibs to your individual taste.
- Each nurse on day duty will report every day at 7 A.M. and leave at 8 P.M. except the Sabbath on which day you will be off from 12 noon to 2 P.M.
- Graduate nurses in good standing with the Director of Nurses will be given an evening off each week for courting purposes, or two evenings a week if you go regularly to church.
- Each nurse should lay aside from each payday a goodly sum of her earnings for her benefits during her declining years so that she will not become a burden. For example, if you earn $30.00 a month, you should set aside $15.00.
- Any nurse who smokes, uses liquor in any form, gets her hair done at a beauty shop or frequents dancehalls will give the Director of Nurses good reason to suspect her worth, intentions, and integrity.
- The nurse who performs her labors, serves her patients and doctors faithfully and without fault for a period of five years, will be given an increase by the hospital administration of $.05 a day, providing there are no hospital debts that are outstanding.

Figure 2–3 The lot of the nurse in 1887

Dorothea Dix (1802–1887)
Instrumental in improving mental hospitals. Volunteer nurse in Civil War, became Superintendent of Women Nurses (first U.S. Army Nurse Corps).

Clara Barton (1821–1912)
Volunteered in Civil War, took other volunteers to battlefield hospitals. Formed American Association of Red Cross and was its first president.

Linda Richards (1841–1930)
First trained nurse in America. Developed nurses' notes. Superintendent of Massachusetts General Hospital School of Nursing. Took nursing education to Japan, 1887.

Mary Eliza Mahoney (1845–1926)
First black professional nurse in America. Worked in private duty. Worked for acceptance of black nurses.

Isabel Hampton Robb (1860–1910)
Nursing educator. Advocated licensure. First nurse to combine career and marriage.

Mary Adelaide Nutting (1858–1947)
Raised standards of nursing education. Reduced students' hours to 8-hours a day.

Lillian D. Wald (1867–1940)
Beginning of public health nursing, emphasized quality of home care.

Clara Maass (1876–1901)
Served with U.S. Army in Spanish American War. Volunteered as test subject in 1901 in experiments with mosquitoes and yellow fever. Only American and only woman to die in the experiment. Honored by the U.S. Postal Service with a commemorative stamp in 1976.

Lydia Hall (–1969)
Concern for nursing care beyond acute stage of illness. Initiated nurse-operated health care facility (Loeb Center for Nursing and Rehabilitation).

Elizabeth Kenny (1886–1952)
Australian nurse who brought innovative ideas for the treatment of poliomyelitis to the United States in 1933.

Figure 2–4 Some leaders of American nursing

> **Esther Lucile Brown**
> Nursing researcher, reported functions performed by nurses. Her 1970s reports form the basis for changes in nursing.
>
> **Hilda Torrop**
> First executive director of the Association of Practical Nurse Schools, now the National Association of Practical Nurse Education and Services.
>
> **Mildred Montag**
> Nursing educator whose work led to the development of community college nursing programs.
>
> **Luther Christman**
> Practitioner, administrator, educator, researcher. Goal is to continue improvement of clinical practice.
>
> **Virginia Henderson**
> Defined nursing as a unique realm of health care, assisting individuals in meeting the basic needs of daily living. Improved nursing library resources.
>
> **Reva Rubin**
> Among leaders in maternal-child health. Instrumental in introducing natural childbirth and rooming-in.

Figure 2-4 (Continued)

survival rates. Complicated injuries could be successfully treated. The fragmentation of medicine into specializations was accelerated. One example was the refinement of plastic surgery to repair disfiguring trauma.

The need for nurses near the battlefields left the people at home without enough nurses; this led to the growth of many *ancillary workers* in health care. Ancillary workers included technicians, nursing assistants, and volunteers; many of these were not originally licensed for their work. In 1943, the Federal government began funding some nursing programs in order to increase the number of nurses.

Advanced medical skills, developed to treat wartime casualties, became useful in civilian practice. Injuries from automobile accidents or fingers amputated from a corn-picking machine were similar to wartime trauma. These advances and the growing population led to increased use of hospitals after the War, and in 1946, the Hill-Burton Act became law. This granted $900 million to local communities for the construction of hospitals. Many present-day small community hospitals had their beginnings then. Hill–Burton hospitals were supposed to contribute 4.4 percent of their beds as free care to people who could not afford it otherwise.

The Vocational Education Act of 1948 was intended to help return veterans back into the work world. One of its provisions led to the rapid increase of programs to educate practical nurses in vocational schools. Registered nurse education also continued to expand in hospitals. There was a need for more nurses to staff the growing number of hospitals. Nurses were primarily generalists, trained to give personal care to hospitalized patients and to assist the physicians with technical procedures such as beginning intravenous fluids.

The Joint Commission on Accreditation of Hospitals (JCAH) was established in 1951. This is a voluntary organization which oversees hospital policies and establishes regulations. Its primary function is to insure the quality of patient care.

More scientific growth accompanied the Korean Conflict. M.A.S.H. units functioned close to the battlefields, demonstrating that rapid treatment of critical injuries could save many lives. This led to growth of more sophisticated emergency care in hospitals.

Two-year nursing programs began in community colleges. In 1956 there were 25 programs. These programs did not require students to be single or to live in dormitories, so they were attractive to many students.

The Later Years (1960–1988) The population continued to grow and health care remained a priority concern. Research into the causes of problems expanded. For example, the polio virus was discovered and a vaccine developed for the prevention of polio. Space technology had major effects on medicine and health care. Examples are the use of computers, microsurgery, and lasers. Transplants of major organs, such as kidneys and hearts, became familiar procedures. Machinery to support life during lengthy surgery increased surgeons' capabilities to try more and more complex procedures.

The Vietnam Conflict contributed to health care by demonstrating the use of jet helicopters for rapid transfer of the severely injured. This concept was soon adapted to civilian hospitals.

As technology increased, health care became more specialized and more expensive. There were shortages of doctors, so nurses were expected to do more. Soon there was a shortage of nurses as well. Nurses were required to take care of the equipment as well as the patients. More workers were needed, not only in number but also in kind. Additional skilled persons were employed to manage the equipment: respiratory therapists and technicians, surgical technicians, electrocardiographic technicians, electroencephalographic technicians, and many others.

Programs in nursing education also changed to meet changing needs. Nurses studied planning and management as well as technical skills. Nursing programs in junior and community colleges grew. These two-year programs often replaced three-year programs which hospitals found too expensive to continue. During this period licensure of nurses became mandatory in all states.

Baccalaureate nursing education also grew rapidly. Some innovative programs were developed to assist nurses achieve higher degrees as well. Today it is not unusual to meet nurses with Master's or Doctoral Degrees. Table 2–1 summarizes the development of nursing education in the United States.

Paying for the care of dependent people, especially the elderly and the disabled, is becoming a major concern as this century moves toward its close. In 1980 the percentage of the population over the age of 65 was 11 percent. Demographers predict that number will double between the years 2000 and 2030. There will continue to be a great need for nurses.

The history of health care from the early 1800s to the present decade is condensed in Table 2–2.

KEY CONCEPT: HISTORICAL REVIEW

- Health care was based on need and ability to pay.
- Most care was given in homes until hospitals became safe and popular—after 1900.
- Nursing education was started in hospitals, then moved into vocational schools and colleges.
- Technology developed in war times helped to advance medical care.
- The government became more involved in health care.

LEVELS OF INTERVENTION

Factors which make up each level of health care intervention are listed in figure 2–5 on page 26. Nurses are actively involved in all four levels: health promotion, primary prevention, curative intervention and maintenance and rehabilitation.

Table 2-1 Evolving nursing education in the United States

YEARS	DEVELOPMENT
1800–1850	Nurses learned by experience. Short training period for some Catholic Sisters. Many practical nurses worked in homes.
1861	Women's Hospital of Philadelphia began six-month training program.
1873	Three hospital-based training programs.
1875	"Nurses' caps" invented.
1885	34 hospital-based training programs, 1–2 years.
1892	Brooklyn YWCA began Ballard School for Practical Nurses.
1893	47 hospital-based training programs.
1903	First licensing of nurses.
1909	Beginning of collegiate programs for nurses.
1914	First state law for practical nurse education.
1923	Hospital programs agreed on 28 month program.
1943	Registered nursing education receives federal funds.
1948	Vocational education funds help practical nurse education.
1956	Beginning of two-year college programs for nurses. (25)
1964	Nurse Training Act stimulated development of baccalaureate and graduate programs in nursing.
1965	Beginning of advanced education for Nurse Practitioners. ANA proposes two levels of nursing: professional and technical.
1971	California passed first mandatory law for continuing education. Many states followed the trend.
1978	ANA supports career mobility.
1980	697 two-year college programs.
1982	NLN supports career ladder opportunities.
1986	North Dakota establishes two levels of nursing education: baccalaureate degree for professional practice (RN); associate degree for technical practice (LPN).

Table 2–2 Summary of United States health care history

YEARS	SOCIETY	HEALTH CARE
1800–1850	Home and family Agricultural Settling the West	Self-help Few doctors or hospitals Poor Houses
1850–1900	Civil War Beginning industrialization	Home-based Hospitals started Doctors licensed Few nurse training programs
1900–1940	More industry World War I Depression Social Security programs	More use of hospitals Hospital schools of nursing Government programs for mothers, children
1940–1988	World War II Growing technology Korean Conflict Space Age Vietnam Conflict Longer lifespan	Antibiotics developed Medical specializations Growing health care industry More government rules Transplants Ethical problems

Level I: Health Promotion

This level focuses on preserving and protecting the population. Health workers try to enhance the health of society at large. In other words, we want to meet the basic human needs of hygiene, safety, food, and shelter.

It is believed that people in industrialized countries have longer life expectancies. This is not because of technology and medication. It is because the people in those countries understand the importance of adequate nutrition and cleanliness to prevent infection and the spread of disease.

In the United States, health is promoted primarily through regulations and education. Federal regulations promote general health. For example, the Environmental Protection Agency monitors the quality of the air, soil, and water.

Americans are educated to promote their own health through campaigns against smoking, alcohol consumption, and the abuse of other chemicals. Drivers of motor vehicles are taught to be on the defensive. Foods are advertised as being "good for you"; even restaurants are serving low-calorie, low-salt meals. Keeping physically fit has become an industry.

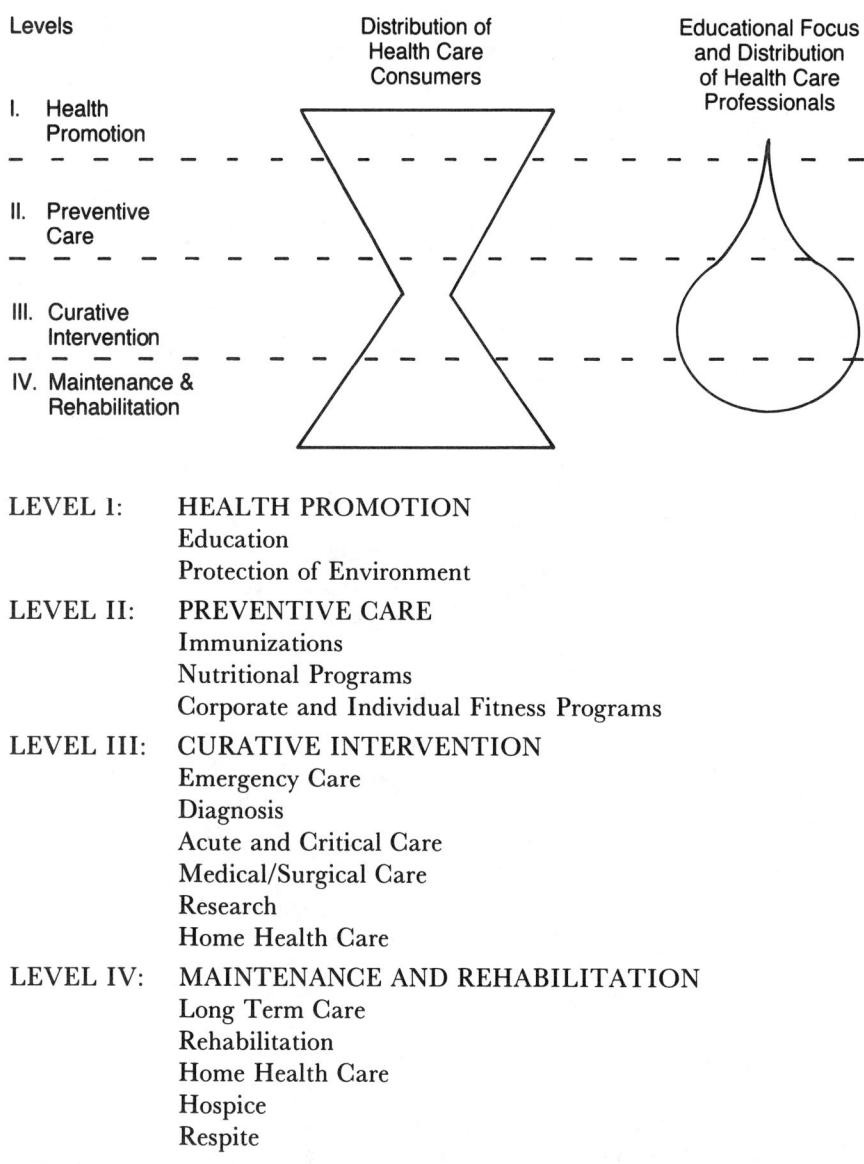

LEVEL I:	HEALTH PROMOTION
	Education
	Protection of Environment
LEVEL II:	PREVENTIVE CARE
	Immunizations
	Nutritional Programs
	Corporate and Individual Fitness Programs
LEVEL III:	CURATIVE INTERVENTION
	Emergency Care
	Diagnosis
	Acute and Critical Care
	Medical/Surgical Care
	Research
	Home Health Care
LEVEL IV:	MAINTENANCE AND REHABILITATION
	Long Term Care
	Rehabilitation
	Home Health Care
	Hospice
	Respite

Figure 2–5 Levels of health care compared with use and health care professionals

Nurses may participate in health promotion (Level I) by being role models and resource persons in their communities. Perhaps you've already been asked by a relative to explain a low-sodium diet. Neighbors feel free to ask nurses questions to decide if the problem requires a doctor's attention. Nurses must be aware of their influence in this area.

Level II: Primary Prevention

This level of health care intervention is a more direct approach to prevent specific problems in certain populations. Community health has always been concerned with prevention and control of disease.

Immunization programs are a good example of primary prevention. Infants and preschoolers are routinely immunized for diphtheria and tetanus; in many states, children must be immunized for measles before they can enroll in public school. Elderly people are encouraged to have flu shots every autumn. In disaster situations, whole populations are often immunized against cholera or typhoid. Nurses often serve as volunteers for these programs. The American Red Cross employs nurses to coordinate preventive programs.

Nutritional programs are also aimed at preventing illness among certain populations. School lunch and breakfast programs were initiated to ensure that children would have adequate meals. Title III of the Older Americans Act provides for subsidized meals for persons over 60; congregate dining centers and meals-on-wheels are tangible examples. The Women, Infant and Children Program (WIC) assists low-income pregnant or nursing women to buy quality foodstuffs for themselves and their young children. The use of food stamps and the WIC program have proven to be cost effective in saving children from serious health problems. Studies suggest that every dollar spent on WIC saves three dollars in the first year on the health care of children who might otherwise be born prematurely or with low birth weight.

Employers have begun programs to prevent health problems for their employees. Large corporations have built gymnasiums, running tracks, or swimming pools for the use of their employees during lunch breaks or before or after work. It is predicted that 25 percent of large corporations will have developed fitness programs by 1991. Some offer bonuses for weight loss; others provide classes to help people break their smoking habits. Occupational health nurses often coordinate such programs. Some companies have hired nurses to teach wellness programs.

Level III: Curative Intervention

This level of health care delivery uses more money than any other level. Curative intervention is defined as treating with the intent to cure, or to prevent death. It remains the major emphasis of research today. By late 1984, the amount of $200 million had been spent on developing the artificial heart. This does not include costs following implantation. Since issues about quality and length of life continue following such surgery, the cost of this technology is still in question.

Medicine and most of health care focused on curative intervention until the early 1980s. Cures are often dramatic and provide much satisfaction. The emphasis on this curative aspect has created the health care industry as it is known today. This health care industry with its hospitals and long term care facilities, employs the greatest number of nurses, as well as technicians and other workers.

Nursing education has focused primarily on curative intervention. Nurses were needed in this area of health care to help the physicians. Present and future nursing practice requires a high degree of technical expertise because of high technology developments.

Level IV: Maintenance and Rehabilitation

Health care intervention at this level deals with chronic conditions and living with disabilities. The technology which helped advance Level III (curative intervention) resulted in greater numbers of consumers in Level IV. Curative medicine can save the life of the stroke victim who then will need rehabilitation services and other support. Technology can save very premature infants; as a result, they may live with multiple disabilities. Longer life spans mean that more people live to go through the normal aging processes; this means that they may develop degenerative joint disease, hypertension or coronary artery disease.

Trauma victims from wartime or peacetime now live as paraplegics or quadraplegics; technology at the scene of injury saves many lives. These people want to live as normally as possible, but they need some kind of health maintenance and social services in order to do so.

The growing number of consumers in this area causes strain on the facilities and services available. The costs of this care are enormous. Basic care in many long term care facilities is about $1500–$2000 per month, and this does not include medications or special therapies. Because more money was previously spent educating workers for Level III, we lack sufficient personnel educated to help with maintenance and rehabilitation. Some changes are happening, however. Research spending on Alzheimer's Disease, for example, has increased almost tenfold since 1976; in 1984 the amount was $37 million.

Nurses have been employed in long term care and rehabilitative facilities. They have very important roles to fill in Level IV and there will be more opportunities as the number of patients in this level will increase.

UNIT 2/HEALTH CARE DELIVERY SYSTEM

More and more of these patients will continue to live at home and need visits from home health care providers. Others will be cared for in still-evolving types of long term care facilities. Nurses are a major resource for these patients and their families.

KEY CONCEPT: LEVELS OF INTERVENTION

- Level I: Health Promotion
- Level II: Primary Prevention
- Level III: Curative Intervention
- Level IV: Maintenance and Rehabilitation

PUBLIC POLICY AND THE HEALTH CARE SYSTEM

The founding fathers came to this country for a quality of life they felt lacking in Europe. Today they might feel that this quality of life is threatened by our health care system; the uneven distribution of health care has resulted in inadequate care for many.

Some people expect the government to help solve problems. Consumers are becoming more vocal in their demands. Special interest groups know how to lobby for their own benefits. In many cases it seems that the government responds only to crisis. Figure 2–6 demonstrates the way some issues have been handled.

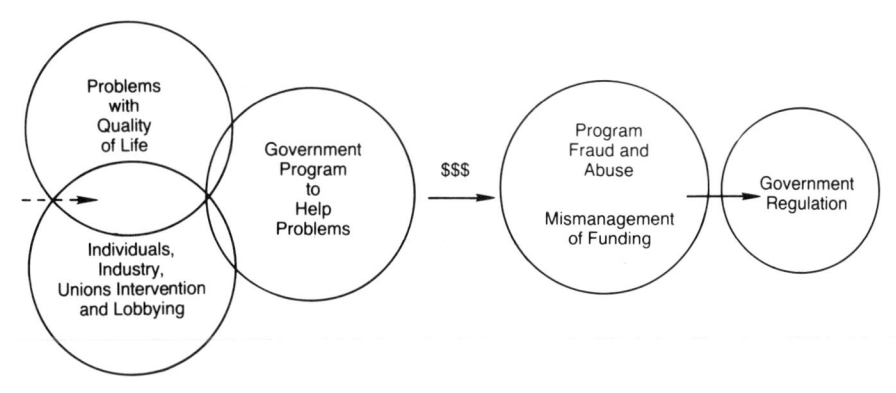

Figure 2–6 A pattern of solving health care problems

Public Policy for a Specific Population

Federal programs have been developed to meet special needs, table 2–3. Changes in the Maternal and Child Health Care Act over the years are an example of the development of public policy. In early 1900 children often worked in factories to supplement the family income. The Children's Bureau was created to protect children and working women. It controlled the number of hours children could work and prevented other abuses.

The Sheppard–Towner Act addressed the nutrition, hygiene, education, and equipment needs for pregnant women. Federal funds were channeled to the states and then to the local governments to provide supplies for home births, among other things. Nurses were employed by county health departments to implement this kind of care.

As part of the recovery program after the Depression, Title V of the Social Security Act provided more federal aid for maternal and child health and medical care for crippled children. It also funded child welfare services. In 1943 the Emergency Maternity and Infant Care Act provided maternity

Table 2–3 Programs developed to meet social needs

YEAR	SOCIAL SCENE	LEGISLATIVE ACTION
1912	Industrialization	Creation of Children's Bureau. Protected children and women from abuses in factories.
1921–1929	Economy poor, economic Depression	Sheppard–Towner Act. Care of pregnant women: nutrition, education, equipment for home births.
1935	Recovery from Depression	Title V, Social Security Act. Funds for maternal and child health, crippled children, child welfare.
1943	World War II	Emergency Maternity and Infant Act. Care of military wives, day care for children.
1963	Technology enables better research	Social Security Amendments. Funds for research: reproduction, growth and development, mental retardation, congenital anomalies.
1964–5	Antipoverty program	Economic Opportunity Act. Neighborhood health centers, more services for maternal and child health.

care for wives of servicemen. It also provided day care for children of working mothers since many women took factory jobs during World War II.

The Social Security Amendments of 1963 provided research funds for the National Institute of Child Health and Human Development. The project was concerned with reproduction, growth and development, mental retardation, and congenital abnormalities.

In 1964, the Economic Opportunity Act (EOA) established the framework for the antipoverty program. It also provided funds for the development of neighborhood health centers. The Social Security Amendments of 1965 allowed grants to states for maternal and child health. Maternity service became more comprehensive. These Acts have since had several revisions; however, the basic purpose remains the same.

National Health Care Problems

The apparent success in providing highly specialized, expensive health care to the majority of our citizens has resulted in several crises for our nation.

- We spend a larger share of the *Gross National Product* (GNP) on health care than any other country—10 percent in 1984. (The GNP is the total amount spent on all goods and services in the country in one year.)
- We are NOT the healthiest nation in the world. In 1985 Chicago physicians reported increasing numbers of cases of *kwashiorkor* and *marasmus*, severe examples of nutritional deprivation among poor children. We are not even in the top ten countries with the lowest infant mortality rates. In 1983 the United States was listed as 12th, with 11.2 deaths per 1000 live births.
- Health care professionals are not evenly distributed. Metropolitan areas and universities with big research centers have more available physicians, facilities and technology than rural areas do.
- Health care knowledge is also unevenly spread among our citizens because of geographical and educational differences.
- The population as a whole has become accustomed to unlimited resources for health care. In 1984, President Reagan appealed for a liver donor for a youngster with biliary atresia; no one mentioned costs. Insurance coverage has insulated the consumer from the true cost of health care.
- Increasing technology has been accompanied by yet unanswered questions about moral and ethical dilemmas. Who should have what transplant? Who will pay for it? When does death occur? When does life begin?

> ### KEY CONCEPT: PUBLIC POLICY FOR HEALTH CARE
>
> - America wants to provide good health care for all its people.
> - Government programs help provide health care for some groups.
> - Many health care problems exist in spite of good intentions and government intervention.

SUMMARY

The growth of health care and its delivery system has paralleled growth in industry and society. There have been spurts in growth when crises such as wars occur. Technology in other sciences has often led to changes in medical and health care as well.

Where do nurses fit in the health care delivery system? Nursing originated as a women's profession. Women were the primary caregivers in the home before nursing was called a profession. Nursing practice followed the practice of medicine in philosophy, technology, and settings, figure 2–7.

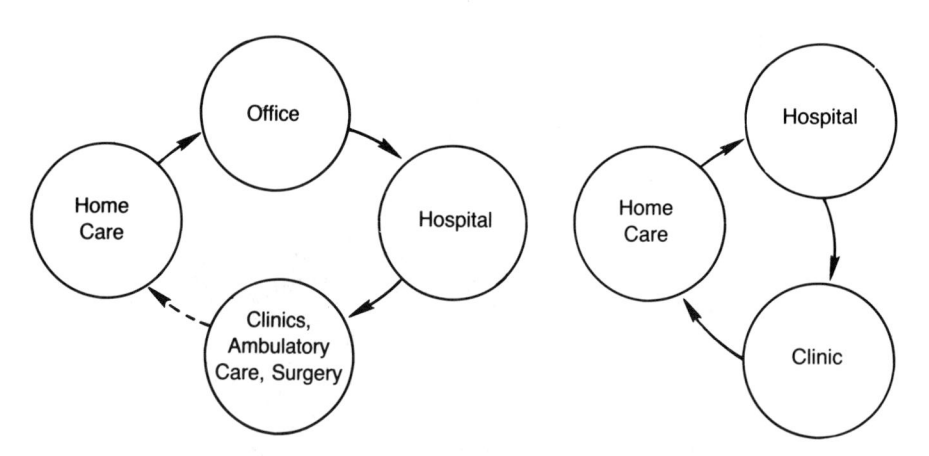

Figure 2–7 Nursing practice followed medical practice in sites of patient care

Nursing has had to change to meet the changing health needs through our history. Employment opportunities have varied with the times. Nursing is beginning to become oriented toward the future instead of just reacting to the changes in health care. Nurses used to do many tasks that doctors delegated to them; now nurses have delegated many functions to technicians and other workers. Nursing organizations are actively involved with legislation to regulate nursing practice and education. However, nurses have not often been actively involved in the total health care delivery system.

Why do problems occur in the system? Much of the answer relates to the shifting political winds. There often seems to be a temporary solution and/or approach to problems. There is a lack of continuity in many policies. Every Congress since 1936 has addressed National Health Insurance in some form, but it has never been passed. The Federal and State governments often disagree on the use of funds. There is no National Health Policy for all citizens.

Why are changes needed? Reviewing this unit should show the need for change. The unequal distribution of care, the skyrocketing costs of health care, and the increasing number of ethical issues beginning to surface are only some of the problems.

Why is it so difficult to change the system? Political structures and regulations, by design, cause change to be a very slow process. There is a lack of public education regarding the total effects of regulations. Some people don't understand how the government works; enacting a law does not necessarily accomplish anything unless funds are also appropriated. And lastly, many cherish the philosophy of Federalism, the preference of local government over a national one.

FOR DISCUSSION

- Identify people you know who are involved in the health care delivery system.
- Is health care a right or a privilege?
- Visit with nurses who practiced in the '50s and '60s. How do they see that nursing has changed?
- Do you think Federalism or Nationalism is the best for health care delivery?
- Pick one of the problems in the health care delivery system. Study how it developed and why it persists. Share your information with your classmates.

QUESTIONS FOR REVIEW

1. List the four parts of the health care delivery system.
2. What philosophy means that local government is supposed to take care of local problems?
3. What was the purpose of the Vocational Education Act of 1948?
4. When did mandatory licensure of nurses become common?
5. List the four levels of health care intervention. Give one example of care given in each level.
6. State the nurse's role in each level of intervention.

3

Paying for Health Care

OBJECTIVES:

After completing this unit, you will be able to:

- Define *fee–for–service* and *prepayment* methods.
- Discuss why cost containment is a health care issue.
- Explain how cost containment has changed health care delivery.
- Identify concerns about payment for health care received in nontraditional settings.

This unit will explain how we pay for health care in the United States. There is no standard method because we believe in individual rights, and because local government is supposed to take care of local needs. Basic alternatives and the development of cost containment programs will be discussed. How payment alternatives and cost containment efforts might affect health care delivery will be examined. Nurses need to have a basic understanding of economics in order to successfully compete in the future. *Economics* is the study of the distribution of resources for goods or services. How is the health care dollar divided for the services needed by our population?

PAYMENT ALTERNATIVES

There are two basic alternatives: the fee–for–service method, and the prepayment method. In the early years doctors were paid according to the resources of the patient and often received eggs, chickens, baked goods or a new fence for their efforts. This was true of most professionals in colonial and frontier days. As the country grew, money rather than goods became the exchange for services. Still, many physicians only charged what they felt the patient could afford, and someone in serious need of care was seldom denied.

The women who nursed the sick rarely received payment beyond their room and board while they worked and helped in the home. When nurses became formally trained, they began to receive small salaries from the doctors or hospitals who employed them, or from the family of the home care patient. The wages were very low, but nurses in hospitals also received room and board (only single women worked in hospitals), uniforms, and one day off each week.

In 1900 the American government was quite decentralized and had little concern for social welfare. A few unions and societies of European immigrants provided their members with a type of insurance for sickness. These plans usually paid the worker for "sick time" rather than hospital or doctor bills. The Granite Cutters Union was first with this benefit in 1877.

Health insurance as it is known today was nearly nonexistant before the 1930s. A few private industries provided direct health service to their employees. In 1914, for example, Metropolitan Life Insurance provided disability insurance to their office employees. Such plans were limited, however, and only paid unusual kinds of bills to protect the worker from financial disaster. The origin of hospitalization insurance may be traced to Dallas, Texas. In 1929, Baylor University Hospital contracted with 1500 teachers in Dallas. The hospital would provide each teacher with up to twenty-one days of hospital care for $6.00 per teacher per year.

As the country recovered from the Depression, more hospitals began offering similar services to particular groups of workers. By 1940, there were thirty-nine Blue Cross plans in the country with 6 million subscribers; private insurance companies had 3.7 million subscribers.

Insurance for doctor bills originated about the same time. Two physicians in California contracted with the Los Angeles Department of Water and Power for the care of two thousand workers and their dependents. In 1935, they had 12,000 workers and 25,000 dependents; each worker paid $2.69 per month for the insurance.

It was also during and after the Depression that the government began paying hospital and doctor costs for people who were unemployed and in need. There have been many changes in those regulations over the years.

When payment for health care is discussed, there are often several parties involved. The *first party* is the patient. The *second party* is the doctor or care provider. A *third party* is another person or organization who will pay all or part of the expenses. (Third party payer refers to payment by an insurance company or by the government). There is even a *fourth party*, the

UNIT 3/PAYING FOR HEALTH CARE

employer who has paid the insurance company premiums. In 1985, businesses paid over $100 billion for health insurance costs. This amount is more than that paid by the combined federal and state governments.

Initially, the insurance company or government agency required the patient to submit the bill directly and would then reimburse the patient for the expenses. This became such a confusing process that personnel in the physician's or hospital office often agreed to take care of the paperwork. At the present time most accounting departments have specialists whose primary responsibility is handling third party accounts, figure 3–1.

The Federal government, as a third party payer through the Social Security Administration, introduced Medicare and Medicaid Insurance plans in 1965. These plans were initially opposed by the American Medical Association (AMA) as they feared it would lead to socialized medicine. The Medicare portion was designed to provide health care for the elderly, many

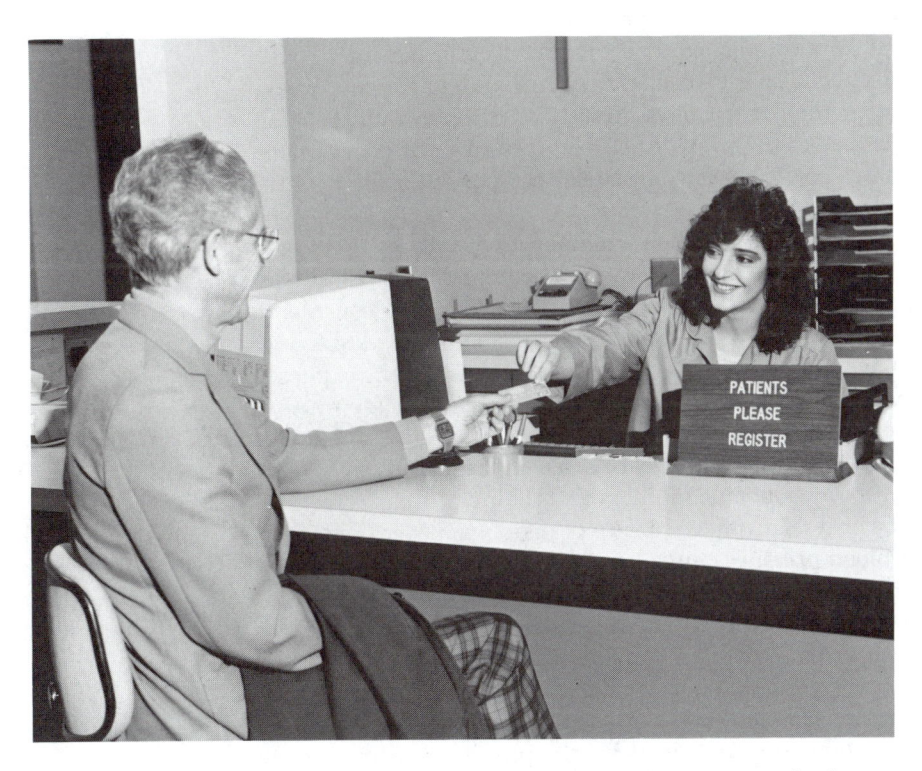

Figure 3–1 Patient presents his insurance card in the computerized payment system.

of whom had never been included in group health insurance during their working years. These people found that they needed more health care as they aged. Often, inflation made costs so great that life savings could easily be threatened by a lengthy illness.

A *means test* requires the person to have an annual income below a certain level to qualify for benefits. There is no means test for Medicare coverage as long as the person is over 65.

Medicaid Insurance does require a means test. It was intended to provide health care to the needy and indigent. Medicaid funds are channeled through the individual states for administration; each state establishes regulations for their distribution.

Fee–for–Service Payments

Fee–for–service is the traditional payment method; services are provided and the patient is billed. Americans pride themselves on paying for goods and services. Private physicians established their practices on the fee–for–service plan. Clinics and hospitals also established accounting departments based on this system. Whether the patient pays directly or through a third party payer makes no difference to the provider. If the insurance or government payment does not match the charges completely, the patient must pay the difference.

The fee–for–service system has been extended to group practices and also covers extended services such as laboratory fees and the use of equipment. The consumer remains quite illness-oriented and rarely consults a doctor unless a problem is suspected. Despite the urging of the AMA and others, few persons have thorough annual physicals because of the expense. Until recently, very few fee–for–service insurance plans paid for routine physical exams or screening procedures.

Public agencies involved in health care often provide *screening services* and clinics, especially for low–income mothers and their children. Screening services are interviews or tests given to a group of people in order to identify certain problems. A blood pressure clinic is one common example. In many situations the patient is still expected to contribute something toward the services rendered; this is called a *sliding-scale* fee schedule.

The patient who visits and pays the same physician for each office visit often develops rapport with that doctor. The patient trusts the physician to control the health care service needed. Most third party payers will not pay for services unless they are prescribed by the physician. Most nurses are employees of doctors, clinics, or institutions. Nursing salaries are included in general costs, they are not paid directly by third party payers. In some states, nurse specialists such as nurse midwives, psychiatric nurse practitioners and pediatric nurse practitioners may receive third party payment without requiring a physician's referral, but this is not yet true nationwide.

The fee–for–service system has been accused of being discriminatory, as it is possible for those with more money to receive more services.

Prepayment Plans

The purpose of prepaid health insurance plans is to prevent illness and maintain wellness. *Health Maintenance Organizations* (HMOs) are examples of prepaid health insurance. The objective is to keep patients healthier by: (1) encouraging regular exams, leading to earlier disease detection, and (2) promoting health education. HMOs grew rapidly during the 1970s.

The essential ingredient for an HMO is a large patient population who pays a fixed amount monthly and then receives ALL necessary health care. Because the emphasis is on preventive health care, patients are encouraged to visit the HMO often. It is less expensive to prevent illness through teaching and care of small problems than it is to treat major illnesses requiring lengthy hospitalizations. A diabetic who is taught to monitor blood sugar and encouraged to call or visit the HMO regularly is less apt to develop a serious complication. The HMO also cares for their patients during times of illness.

In this system, the physicians are employees of the HMO and are salaried along with the other health care workers. They receive the same salary whether they see five or fifty patients in one day. Nurses are employed in these clinics. Independent nurse practitioners and other professionals such as physical therapists and psychologists may also be employed by the HMO and have their own patients. Most HMOs are managed by persons trained in business operatons; they are operated for profit.

HMOs were initially meant for employed persons and their families. When developers of the plan realized that the elderly population needed many services as well, they modified the system so they could accept Medicare patients, too. The elderly pay a small monthly fee for the comprehensive services available. This fixed fee covers the difference between the amount allowed by Medicare and that charged by the HMO. For example, if a patient needs to have a blood cholesterol taken, the HMO may charge $22 but Medicare may pay only $20.

The HMO system of payment has increased competition among physicians, especially in large cities where many HMOs have been organized. The subscriber to an HMO agrees to only use the doctors, clinics, and hospitals which belong to that HMO group. If a specialist is needed for a particular problem, the HMO will decide what specialist the patient should see. The patient may choose other health care professionals, but the cost will have to be paid by the patient.

Combination Plans

In the 1980s, *Preferred Provider Organizations* (PPOs) appeared in some parts of the country. These are a combination of HMOs and the traditional fee-for-service insurance. They are organized much like HMOs. The major difference is that a patient who wants to see a specialist who does not belong to the plan may do so; the PPO will pay a percentage of the fee.

There are new forms of health insurance being developed and marketed across the country. Some of them are for only certain groups, considered to be good risks. Consumers can easily become confused about the varieties of coverages available.

Issues Regarding Payment Plans

Paying for health care remains a problem. There are critics of every method, none of which has successfully held the line on inflationary costs. Much of the public remains concerned only with illness, and many do not take advantage of health education or preventive medicine.

Americans have developed a new awareness of health, however, and are taking more responsibility for their own health. People have become more assertive and less passive as discriminating consumers of health care services. Education encourages consumers to keep trim and fit, exercise regularly, and eat in moderation. Health needs of specific groups are more clearly identified. Elderly people often have chronic health problems. Many executives have stress-related disorders.

Consumerism also affects health care. Community committees and boards for public health programs usually include several members who are consumers of health services. There is better communication between health professionals and the lay public.

A grass-roots effort to improve health services without raising costs is called the *ombudsman* concept. The ombudsman is a person who is politically and financially independent of government, and whose job is to investigate complaints and assist consumers in dealing with government bureaucracy. This effort is intended to truly protect the public. To date, ombudsmen programs have not been popular because agencies prefer self-regulation and fear loss of control.

The Board on Aging has developed a very active ombudsman program in Minnesota. In 1984, seven regional ombudsmen handled 1482 cases related to long term care. Two-thirds dealt with entry into nursing homes and alternative care, and one-third dealt with complaints. Ombudsmen also made educational presentations to groups regarding choosing and financing long term care, rights and responsibilities of nursing home residents and the nursing home regulatory system. A National Ombudsman Association was organized in October, 1984.

> ### *KEY CONCEPT: PAYMENT ALTERNATIVES*
>
> - Fee–for–service is a major alternative; those without money may receive free care.
> - Focus is often on illness care.
> - Prepayment plans have gained popularity since the 1970s. The focus is on preventive care.
> - Controversy about payment plans continues due to the rising costs of health care.

COST CONTAINMENT

Ever since World War II, health care delivery has been a growing industry. Technological advances are expensive, and the patient pays the bills. Patients expect the "best"; physicians and hospitals are happy to oblige.

Many people were unaware of the increasing costs because of insurance payments. Health care workers were not made aware of the costs of supplies or encouraged to be careful with their use. Perhaps only two gauze dressings were needed, but the only package available contained ten; well, that was all right, the ones not used were thrown out. After all, the insurance paid the bills.

Professional Standard Review Organizations (**PSRO**) were established in 1972 by the Social Security Amendments. The intent was to evaluate services provided by Medicare, Medicaid, and Maternal and Child Health Programs. The quality and quantity of health care delivered in acute and long term care facilities was evaluated according to review plans written by doctors and administrators. The goal was to monitor health care so that those in need received quality care for the money spent.

Health care costs continued to escalate in spite of these measures. Inflation in health care services increased by over 12 percent in 1982, a year when the general economy had an inflation rate of a minus 3.9 percent. Figure 3–2 illustrates the percentage of the gross national product (GNP) spent on health care during the past years as well as projections for the immediate future. In 1985, $1 billion was spent each day for health care. That was over $42 million every single hour!

Fee–for–service and assorted insurance plans have been called *retrospective* reimbursement, the bills are paid after the service has been received.

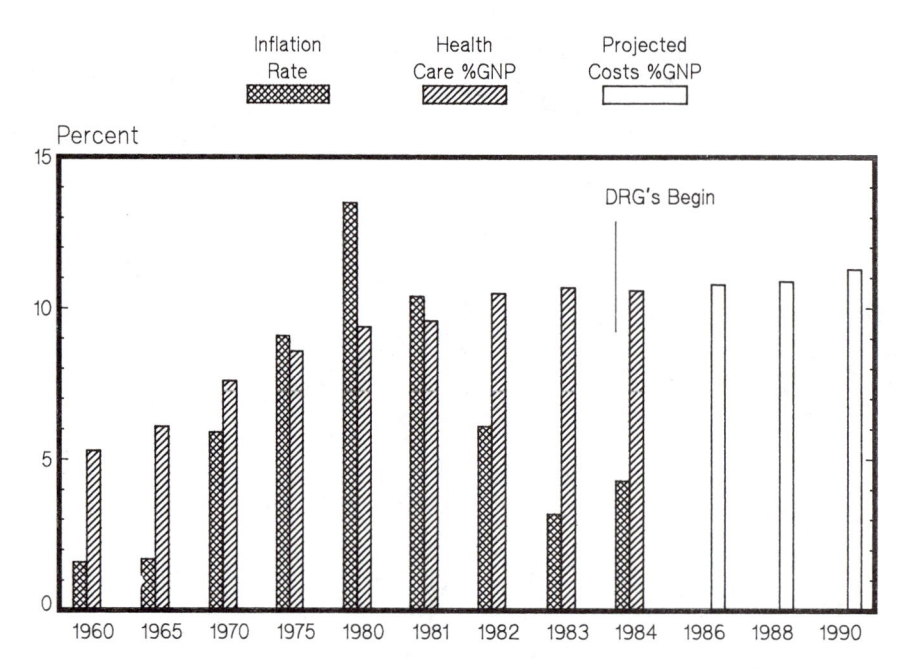

Figure 3-2 Inflation in Health care costs (Data Source: Health Care Financing Administration, U.S. Department of Commerce, Bureau of the Census)

Many authorities say that this type of arrangement has led to a loss of accountability by all involved. It has been compared to a parent giving an adolescent a credit card and agreeing to pay the bills later.

Medicare's Prospective Payment Plan   *HCFA*

The Health Care Financing Administration designed a *Prospective Payment Plan* (PPP) for Medicare patients, which became a law in 1983. Under this plan, commonly referred to as DRGs, Medicare payment for a hospital admission is based on a fixed amount determined in advance according to one of 473 *Diagnostic Related Groups* (DRGs). It replaced the previous fee–for–service payment method used by Medicare. A sampling of DRG classifications is shown in table 3–1.

For example, Mrs. Anderson, aged 70, needs a cholecystectomy and Medicare is going to help pay for it. According to the DRG system, approximately $3500 is allowed for a cholecystectomy performed in a midwestern hospital. If Mrs. Anderson is otherwise quite healthy and recovers rapidly,

UNIT 3/PAYING FOR HEALTH CARE

Table 3–1 Sample DRGs

DRG Number	Code*	Classification**	Diagnosis
6	1	S	Carpal tunnel release
15	1	M	Transient ischemic attacks
44	2	M	Acute major eye infections
59	3	S	Tonsillectomy and/or adenoidectomy age > 17
88	4	M	Chronic obstructive pulmonary disease
107	5	S	Coronary bypass (w and w/o catheterization)
146	6	S	Rectal resection age > 69
235	8	M	Fractures of femur
294	10	M	Diabetes age > 36
336	12	S	Transurethral prostatectomy age > 69 and/or dx 2

*Coded by body systems
**Medical or Surgical diagnostic classification

she may be discharged on the third post-operative day and the hospital bill may be $3100. However, if Mrs. Anderson develops a wound infection and stays in the hospital for six days, the bill may climb to $4200. In either case, Community Hospital receives $3500 Medicare payment. Payments under specific DRG categories do vary in different areas of the country and in urban and rural communities. It is generally agreed that the length of hospitalization has shortened since the implementation of Medicare's DRGs. Table 3–2 demonstrates major differences in the most common payment systems.

Additional Cost Controls

Although DRGs only affect Medicare patients at this time, there is a noticeable "trickle-down" effect as doctors and hospitals become more aware of controlling costs. Fewer hospital admissions are ordered, and all patients are encouraged to leave the hospital as soon as possible. Use of hospital beds is down to 1.8 per 1000 population in many areas of the country.

Many insurance companies have initiated cost containment programs, too. Examples of these efforts include the need for a second opinion before having elective surgery, requiring prior approval of the insurance company before entering the hospital, and allowing independent review of subscriber's charts.

The development of one-day surgery departments and 24 hour discharge of well mothers and newborns are further examples within the industry to limit costs. The prolific growth of home health care can be directly related to cost containment efforts in hospitals.

KEY CONCEPT: NEED FOR COST CONTAINMENT

- Growth in the health care industry creates higher costs. Consumers are often unaware of the total costs because of insurance payments.
- Medicare regulations created DRGs in 1983, specifying amounts payable to hospitals for the care of Medicare patients.
- To control costs, insurance companies began restricting payment, requiring second opinions, etc.
- Cost containment efforts result in shorter hospital stays.

EFFECTS OF COST CONTAINMENT

Traditional Care

The goal of cost containment efforts is to control the cost. Third party payers, whether insurance companies or government agencies, are motivated by economics. Employers who pay the insurance bills are demanding that the cost of benefits be lowered. Many industries claim that too much of their money goes for employee health benefits. The health care industry is, therefore, forced to control expenses.

Patients, as consumers of health care, want to control costs, but not by sacrificing the quality of their own health care. Patients continue to expect the best and most expensive treatment, but the industry is operating on a tight budget.

Table 3-2 Comparison of Payment Methods

	Fee-for-service	HMO	DRG
Clients	Anyone	Subscribers, dependents	Age 65+
Amount paid	Actual costs, patient may have to pay portion	Membership Fee	Fixed rate Hospital only, Medicare
Length of treatment	Unlimited, as needed	Audited by HMO	Federal standards
Who pays	Insurance Company or patient	HMO	Medicare
Incentives for cost containment	None	Prevent problems	Efficient use of services

To many health professionals, cost has always been an unmentionable word. Nurses and doctors who were educated to provide the best of care regardless of expense become frustrated by current demands to limit costs. Many predicted that DRGs would result in poor quality of care; however, no statistical evidence of negative effects due to the DRG regulations has been established to date.

In acute care settings, cost containment has resulted in shorter stays for all types of patients. Surgical patients are expected to do most of their recovery at home; sometimes this means they are taught to change dressings, empty catheter drainage bags, and manage their own pain control regimen. Many patients are capable of learning these skills; individual learning patterns must be considered. Families are included in the teaching and expected to become primary caregivers in many instances.

Another effect in hospitals is that people who are hospitalized are acutely ill, not just "sick." In the 1960s, patients often were admitted for diagnostic tests or for observation until a diagnosis could be determined. Cost containment makes that practice obsolete. As technology increases, more critical patients are maintained on respirators and other devices, stretching the capacity of Intensive Care Units. The less critical patients are more quickly transferred to medical or surgical units, where their complex care is continued. Nurses have to be expert caregivers to manage the care of these patients.

These changes in hospitalization have also affected the long term care facility. Residents are returned from the hospital after acute illness in an improved but still sick state. This requires advanced skills of the long term care nurses to care for very ill residents. More patients also spend some time in long term care facilities for their convalescence before being able to return to their own homes. Medicare funding of long term care is quite restrictive, and many private health insurance companies will not cover long term care at all. Who will pay for extended and long term care in the future?

Nontraditional Care

Early discharge from hospitals has resulted in increased need for home health care. Although this segment of health care delivery has been in existence for over 100 years, it has only recently returned as an adjunct to more traditional care in hospitals. There is much opportunity in this area for nurses. Because the growth of this part of the delivery system is rapid and uncoordinated, it has not yet been well defined or regulated.

Payment for home health care depends on the type of care needed. Medicare guidelines are quite explicit; they are summarized in figure 3-3. Some health insurance companies will pay certain home health care expenses, but usually not all of the costs. Care that is considered to be of the maintenance type is usually not covered by insurance. People who need home health care sometimes cannot have it if no one can pay the bill.

Other kinds of nontraditional care, such as group homes for mentally handicapped persons, may not be included in any health insurance except through government funding. Many payment plans are still based on traditional practices.

KEY CONCEPT: COST CONTAINMENT EFFECTS

- Hospital stays are shorter.
- Hospital patients are very sick.
- Greater technical skills are needed by nurses and others.
- Residents in long term care (LTC) need more skilled care.
- The use of home health care has increased.
- The dilemma continues about rising costs and who should pay for the uninsured.

MEDICARE PAYMENT FOR HOME HEALTH CARE

We all know that Medicare coverage is difficult, if not impossible, to figure out. But when it comes to coverage for home health care there are a few simple points to remember:

- Homebound
- Doctor's Order
- Part-time or intermittent skilled care
- Certified home health care provider

All four of these conditions must be met before you can receive Medicare coverage for home health care.

HOMEBOUND. This means that Medicare requires you to be confined to your home. You must need the assistance of another person or an assistive device such as a wheelchair to travel to doctor appointments or other necessary appointments. You may **not** go out for a walk, shopping or on social outings; this may jeopardize your eligibility for Medicare services. Occasional outings, such as once a month or holiday dinners are permitted.

DOCTOR'S ORDER. This means your doctor must write an order stating the reason for your care. He or she must also set up a home health care plan for your nurse or therapist to follow. If your doctor does not feel home health care services are needed, Medicare will not pay for your care.

PART-TIME OR INTERMITTENT SKILLED CARE. Medicare requires that you need the services of one or more of the following: a registered or licensed practical nurse, a physical therapist, or a speech therapist.

The key to remember is that you must need these services only on a part-time or intermittent basis. By part-time, Medicare usually means for two hours or less (a couple of times per week). If you need the continuous or round-the-clock care of a nurse or therapist, Medicare will not pay for these services in your home.

Medicare also does not pay for "custodial" care. Normally patients need to be newly diagnosed, recently discharged from the hospital following an acute hospitalization, or have some new major changes in care,

Figure 3–3 Medicare payment for home health care (Courtesy of *Minnesota Senior Spotlight*, newsletter of the Minnesota Board on Aging, July–August, 1986)

> such as a wound treatment or medication changes. In other words, Medicare will not pay for long term chronic conditions with no recent complications.
> CERTIFIED HOME HEALTH CARE PROVIDER. This means you **must** receive services from a home health care provider who has been given the "stamp of approval" by Medicare. Many home health care providers are not certified and cannot bill Medicare for your services. Be sure to ask if your provider is certified.

Figure 3–3 (Continued)

SUMMARY

Health care is very expensive. Paying for care has been based on fee–for–service for many years. The growth of the health insurance industry insulated consumers from the true costs. Prepayment plans are gaining in popularity, but remain costly.

Cost containment efforts by the Federal government and the private insurance industry have created many recent changes in the system. Whether efforts to control costs are effective remains to be seen.

FOR DISCUSSION

- What kind of health payment plan do you have? Why? Read the fine print to see whether your plan covers home health care or care in a long term care facility. Who would pay those expenses if needed?
- Investigate the cost of health care in your community. Compare the cost of a procedure done in a hospital with the same procedure done in a clinic.
- What evidence of changes in health care delivery do you see within your geographical area?
- Visit with a Medicare coordinator to learn more about DRGs and their effects on hospital use.

QUESTIONS FOR REVIEW

1. Give three examples of efforts at cost containment.

2. How has the length of hospitalization changed since the implementation of DRGs?

3. Define *fee-for-service* and *prepayment*.

4
Expanded Settings for Health Care Delivery

OBJECTIVES:

After completing this unit, you will be able to:

- Discuss changing nursing roles in traditional care settings.
- Define expanded settings.
- Identify four expanded settings for health care delivery in which nurses are employed.
- Explain four factors which will influence the patient's choice of setting.
- Explain the autonomy of nurses in some expanded settings.

Unit 1 examined some projections for future health care delivery in this country. This unit will discuss two ways in which changes are already occurring. One change is the kind of care given in the traditional places: hospitals, doctors' offices, and nursing homes. The other change is the setting, or place where care is received. *Expanded settings* refer to those areas outside of the traditional places, figure 4–1. Decentralization of health care delivery, as stated earlier, means that more care will be given outside of large institutions. One of the reasons for this change is to keep health care affordable.

These expanded settings offer many employment opportunities for nurses who want to practice basic nursing. *Autonomy* is a key word for nurses practicing in many expanded settings of the future. Nurses have to be able to think independently and make decisions. They need to have a good portion of common sense along with their nursing skills and observation techniques. In some settings, co-workers or supervisors are available to give

UNIT 4/EXPANDED SETTINGS FOR HEALTH CARE DELIVERY 51

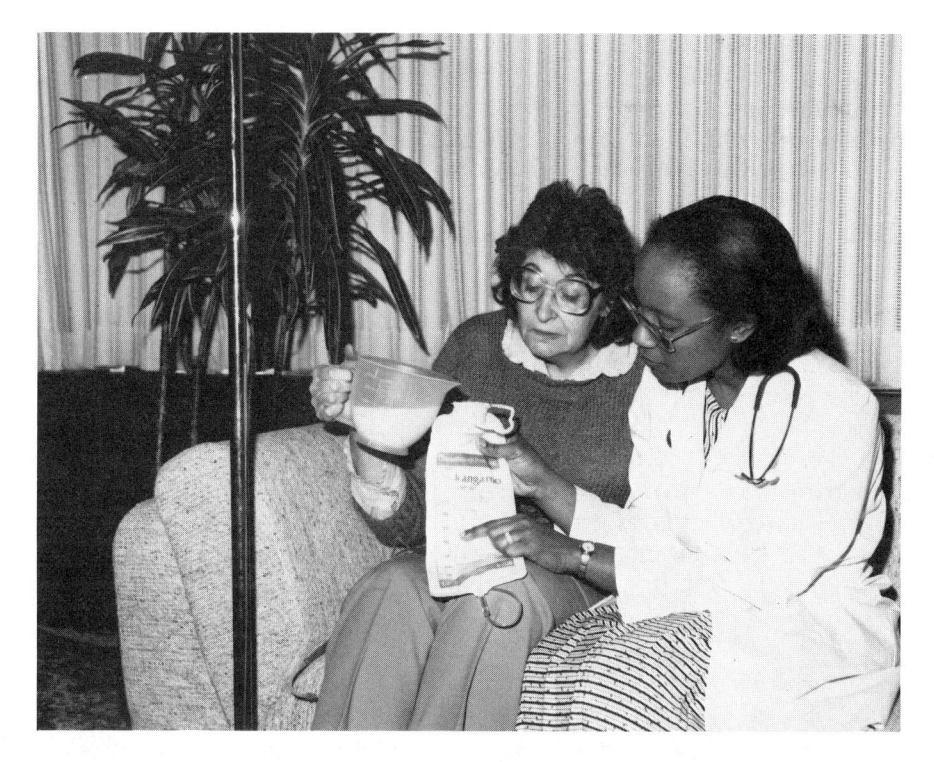

Figure 4-1 Home health nurse supervises a gastrostomy tube feeding.

advice. In other settings, the nurse is alone with the patient. The decisions may have long-lasting effects on the patient, so the nurse must be careful, knowledgeable, and confident. Other changes needed in nursing care will be mentioned only briefly here. The application of basic concepts will be described in much more detail in Unit 10.

CHANGING CARE IN TRADITIONAL SETTINGS

Hospitals

As a general rule most patients in acute care hospitals are very ill. Hospitals are used for major surgery and for acute, complicated problems. The man who needs a bowel resection will be hospitalized for the surgery and the immediate postoperative period. The woman who had a myocardial infarction will be in an Intensive Coronary Care Unit for several days.

The bedside nurse working in a hospital needs special expertise and technical education to manage the care of these very ill patients with the *high tech* equipment. High tech in health care has come to mean the use of computerized monitors and other electronic devices to assist in data collection and patient care. In-service classes are often available, especially when new equipment is introduced. Examples of techniques include managing the kangaroo pump for gastrostomy feedings, or reviewing the sterile techniques required to maintain a Hickman catheter. Usually coronary care classes must be taken before a nurse can be employed in such a highly-specialized area.

The nurse is the vital link between the patient and the machinery in these specialized areas. Remember that the patient attached to that computerized monitor and IV pump is a person—a very important person with anxieties and psychosocial needs as well. It is tempting to enter a patient's room and check the IV tubing, the catheter, the oxygen tubing, or the traction equipment. However, patients have been known to remark how nice it is to have a nurse look at their faces first!

Patients are discharged from hospitals very quickly, as long as no complications develop. The man with the bowel anastomosis may be sent home within a week after surgery. He will need instructions about changing his dressings and how to observe for complications. The woman who had a heart attack may also be discharged by the seventh or eighth day. She may need a home health nurse to monitor her cardiac rehabilitation exercises. Sometimes patients are sent home on intravenous antibiotics, chemotherapy, or hyperalimentation. Others are sent home with open surgical wounds requiring regular irrigation and dressing changes.

Discharge planning has always been a part of patient care, but earlier discharges have increased the importance of this planning. Most hospitals now have forms that must be completed for every patient being discharged. You may have already been involved in this kind of discharge planning if it was necessary to explain diet instructions or medication side effects to a patient before he went home.

Nurses are responsible for identifying those patients who need particular planning in order to continue their recovery at home. Some situations may need referral to the head nurse or the hospital social worker for further evaluation. Going home with a cast or an indwelling catheter can be a high anxiety situation for the patient. Nurses are also responsible for teaching patients and their families how to continue the necessary care. If home care nursing is anticipated, the appropriate agency should be notified as early as possible so that coordination of care can be arranged.

Respite Care

Respite means an interval of temporary rest, especially from work or special duty. In health care, respite means that the regular caregiver has a rest while someone else is responsible for the patient. Perhaps the family member giving the care becomes ill or has other responsibilities that interfere temporarily. For example, Mr. Jones has severe arthritis and and cannot dress or feed himself. His wife manages his daily care quite well. Perhaps Mrs. Jones wants to attend her grandson's wedding in another state; she may arrange respite care for Mr. Jones during her absence. Perhaps she wants someone to visit her husband for a few hours each week while she does their shopping; this could also be considered respite.

Respite care has developed in traditional health care facilities as an alternative use of existing rooms or units. Hospitals can arrange for a certain percentage of their beds to be *swing beds*. These beds can then be used for respite care at times, or "swung" into acute care beds if needed. The designated use of the beds can be changed according to the hospital's needs.

People hospitalized for respite care include the dependent elderly or the handicapped person whose regular caregiver becomes ill, needs a little free time, or is taking a vacation. Respite care provides room and board and minimum aid or supervision with bathing and dressing. The patients or clients often must provide their own medication, which the nurse will administer as the physician orders. The regular staff nurses provide this kind of respite care in the hospital.

Respite care can also be arranged in some traditional nursing home facilities. Sometimes home health care agencies are asked to provide respite care.

Long Term Care

One kind of long term care facilities are those institutions that used to be called "nursing homes." These settings are no longer only used for care of the dependent elderly in our society. They may also be used for the comatose youngster with Reyes' Syndrome, the quadriplegic young adult, and the middle-aged person who is debilitated because of multiple sclerosis. In some settings, these patients may require intravenous therapy, gastrostomy feeding tubes, or tracheostomy suctioning. These therapies require that the nurses in these facilities keep abreast of many technical aids to patient care.

Many long term care facilities also have short term patients who are recovering from surgery or cardiovascular accident (CVA), patients who need several months of care and therapy before resuming independent living. This can be called "extended care."

Changes have occurred because of cost-containment policies in hospitals. Nurses in long term care also need extra education to learn to be leaders, since much of the patient care is given by nursing assistants. Personnel management classes are offered through in-service or adult education programs.

Medical Clinics

A clinic is usually composed of several physicians who share office facilities and work cooperatively. These clinics are also changing in response to greater competition for patients. Many are open for extended hours, including Saturdays, to better accommodate patients. Some clinics also perform many diagnostic tests, such as GI x-rays or gastroscopy, that used to be available only in hospitals. Minor surgical procedures such as myringotomy with tube insertion, laparoscopies, and short term intravenous therapy may also be performed in some clinics, figure 4–2. In figure 4–3, a clinic nurse is administering intravenous chemotherapy.

Nurses employed in these progressive clinics need to be capable of a wide variety of responsibilities. These nurses are truly generalists.

KEY CONCEPT: CARE IN TRADITIONAL SETTINGS CHANGES

- **Hospitalized patients are acutely ill.** Nurses need to understand high tech equipment, but remember the person being treated. Earlier discharge requires more patient education and better discharge planning.
- Respite care may be given in hospitals, nursing homes, and at home.
- **Long term care includes all ages of patients.** Sometimes high tech machinery is used in long term care.
- Traditional medical clinics now offer more services, including some that previously required hospitalization.

NEW SETTINGS FOR ACUTE CARE

Ambulatory Care Centers

Ambulatory centers for acute care are similar to doctors' offices, except that they encourage "walk-ins." Since no appointments are needed, people can get immediate attention and care. Some of these centers are associated with traditional hospitals. Some are even part of a hospital. Others are entirely

Cystoscopy	Chemotherapy Treatment
Gastroscopy	Diagnostic Radiography
Proctoscopy	Myringotomy
Duodenoscopy	Cast Application
Bronchoscopy	Tubal Ligation
Laparoscopy	Vasectomy
Dilatation and Curettage (D & C)	

Figure 4-2 Procedures performed in some clinics today

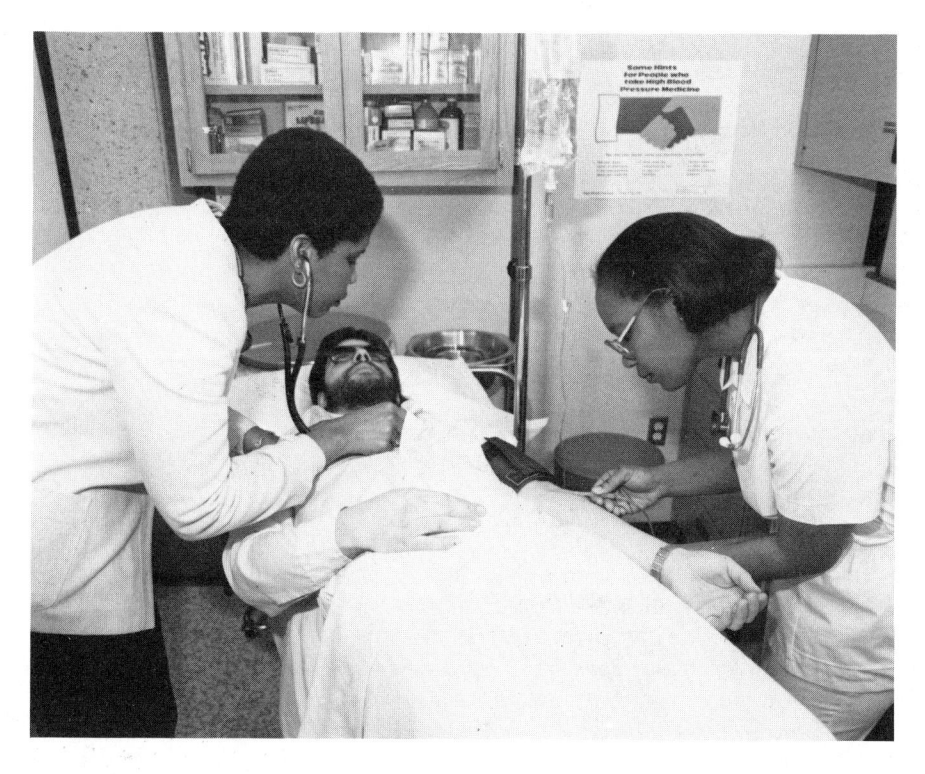

Figure 4-3—Nurse administering intravenous chemotherapy

independent. Some can be found in neighborhoods that would otherwise lack adequate health care.

These care centers call their patients "consumers." They are marketed as being more accessible, quicker, and less expensive than traditional offices and hospital emergency rooms. Many care centers are open 12 to 16 hours, every day including weekends and holidays.

What kinds of health care can be received in an ambulatory care center? Sometimes accident victims arrive, but more often the problems are quite ordinary: respiratory infections, physical exams, minor health concerns. Patients prefer these centers, where available, because they do not have to wait or make an appointment weeks in advance. The centers are also convenient for travelers, and for those who do not have a family doctor.

Nurses employed in ambulatory care centers have to be adaptable because of the wide variety of conditions seen. As these centers gain in popularity, there will be more employment opportunities for nurses and new challenges in nursing practice.

Ambulatory Surgery Centers

Ambulatory surgery centers may be free-standing or be part of a traditional hospital. They are similar to ambulatory care centers, except that patients usually plan ahead to have ambulatory surgery. The primary reason for development of these centers is the effort to contain costs.

In these settings, patients are admitted, receive preoperative care, have surgery, recover, and are discharged all in one day. Many operative procedures may be done in an ambulatory center: herniorrhaphy, cataract extraction, bunionectomy. The nursing care focuses on pre- and postoperative care, and giving the patient more education about recovery care at home. It is obvious that in some situations these centers may be in competition with progressive medical clinics.

Day Care for Ill Children

Not feeling good is part of being a child. There are times when children are too ill to be in school or in regular day care settings, but not ill enough to keep mom or dad home from work. Day care settings specifically for these children is another expanded area of health care delivery. Because most parents in this country are employed outside of the home, the popularity of this kind of facility is growing.

Many of these centers are open year around, especially those in larger cities. Children are observed, medicated, settled for naps, entertained and given lots of TLC, just like at home! Parents are able to continue working, knowing that their child is being cared for by competent persons. The center is also less expensive than hiring a private duty nurse!

A variation of this kind of care center is one that is designed for children with handicaps or chronic conditions such as cerebral palsy or spina bifida. Many such children are regularly cared for in their homes, but parents may need respite time occasionally. It is likely that more of these specialized day care facilities will develop in the future.

✱ **KEY CONCEPT: NEW SETTINGS FOR ACUTE CARE**

- Ambulatory care centers
- Ambulatory surgery centers
- Day care centers for the care of ill children

NEW SETTINGS FOR LONG TERM CARE

Convalescent Care Facilities

Convalescent care facilities are settings for patients who are recovering from major health problems or receiving extensive rehabilitation therapy. These patients are not yet able to care for themselves at home, but are no longer acutely ill. As hospitals focus on the most critical patients, those who are more stable will be transferred to intermediate care.

Some of these facilities are in hospitals, some are in nursing homes, and some are independent settings. An example of a patient who would benefit might be the widowed lady in her early 70s who has had a hip replaced. She was independent before the surgery and will be again, but for a few weeks she will need assistance with daily activities and rehabilitation. Another example would be someone recovering from surgery who needs regular wound irrigations but has no family member to help at home.

Convalescent care facilities employ nurses to work with therapists, give medications, and supervise nursing assistants. Observation skills and the ability to function autonomously are very important.

Community Homes

Some people need a little supervision with their daily lives. Examples of people who may be temporarily served in community homes include those recovering from chemical dependency or mental illness. Other people need a temporary home during a time of crisis, such as battered women and their children or runaway adolescents.

Others need supervision permanently—some mentally handicapped people, some with chronic mental health problems, some with physical disabilities. The handicapped individual is now part of everyday society. Community homes often developed when large institutions were closed. Many are organized by the state or county. Some are private organizations. Most employ nurses to manage medication routines and help with counselling and therapies.

Shared housing for people with slight deficits is another example of community supervision. An apartment building may have four apartments, each with two bedrooms and housing four adults. The people can be "matched" so that one can do light housekeeping, another cook the meals, and another drive. The sixteen people agree to help each other with minimal outside assistance. Perhaps a public health nurse will visit monthly. This model is suggested especially for the elderly who are well but no longer can maintain an individual home and have no family in the community.

Day Care for the Elderly or Disabled Adult

In many areas of the country, nursing homes have added day care facilities to their services, figure 4-4. This arrangement provides a place for dependent elderly persons to stay while their caregiver (spouse, child, neighbor) is employed or away for the day. The facilities provide the noon meal, diversional therapy, a rest period, and companionship. Some also provide transportation services. An example of a day care patient is someone with early Alzheimer's Disease who can still function but needs supervision.

Nurses employed in day care programs are responsible for medication administration, making observations, recordkeeping, and supervising assistants and volunteers. Making sure that families are kept aware of changes in the dependent person's condition is also important. Sometimes a social worker is the case coordinator for adult day care settings.

Hospices

Hospice care is a very specialized kind of care which began in England and came to the United States in the late 1960s. It is still evolving. It is best defined as a philosophy of care in which the quality of the patient's life is the most important consideration while preparing for death. Hospices vary in organizational structure: some are in-patient and part of the hospital; some are in-patient independent facilities; some are entirely based on home

THE CARE COVE
ADULT DAY CARE PROGRAM

When You Need to Set Anchor, But There's No Shore In Sight...

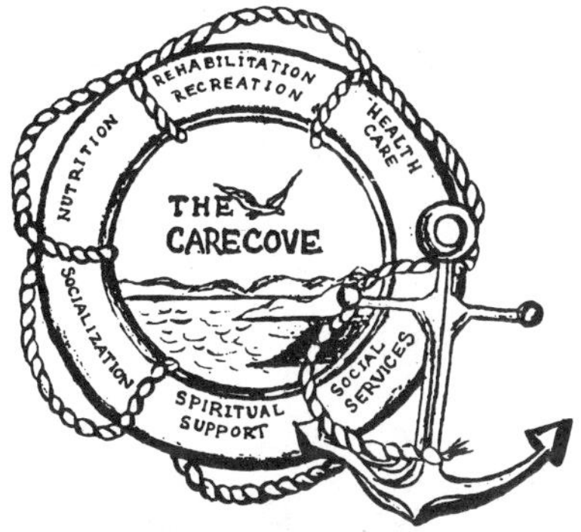

AN ALTERNATE CARE SERVICE

- HEALTH CARE MONITORING
- REHABILITATION
  (OCCUPATIONAL, PHYSICAL, SPEECH, THERAPIES)
- NUTRITION INFORMATION
- SOCIAL SERVICES
- SPIRITUAL SUPPORT
- RELAXATION
- RECREATION
- SOCIALIZATION
- TEMPORARY RELIEF FOR REGULAR CARE GIVERS

Program hours: M-F,
7:30 A.M. - 5:00 P.M.

...COME TO THE CARE COVE

A COMMUNITY SERVICE OF BETHEL HOME OF VIROQUA
VIROQUA, WI 54665

Figure 4–4 Example of Day Care Service (Courtesy of James B. Olson, Administrator of Bethel Home, Viroqua, Wisconsin)

care; some are a combination of in-patient and home care situations. Figure 4–5 lists characteristics of most hospices.

Nurses employed in hospice care need to understand the hospice philosophy as well as their own feelings about death and dying. Basic comfort care needed by hospice patients is the essence of bedside nursing, whether at home or in a separate facility.

The future of hospices is uncertain because of regulatory questions being raised. Agencies often require established time frames and cost analyses as a framework for developing regulations. Since the length of time the person is a hospice patient is uncertain, it is difficult to estimate costs. As a result, hospice care is not covered by all third party payers; some patients who could benefit by hospice care may not be able to afford it.

- Staffed by interdisciplinary team—physicians, nurses, social workers, therapists, clergy, volunteers—working together.
- Patients are admitted for comfort care when cure is no longer possible.
- Entire family is the team's concern.
- Staff is available 24 hours for home care support.
- Bereavement follow-up is included for family and staff.
- Staff continuing education is very important.

Figure 4–5 Characteristics of a hospice

> ✳ **KEY CONCEPT: NEW SETTINGS FOR LONG TERM CARE**
>
> - Convalescent care facilities
> - Community homes
> - Day care for the elderly or disabled adult
> - Hospices

EXPANDED USE OF HOME HEALTH CARE

Health care has always been given in homes, but the recent years have brought about a great increase in organized home health care agencies. This change is primarily due to cost containment efforts and the earlier discharge of patients from hospitals.

Home health care patients include people of all ages and conditions. New mothers and their babies are referred after their 24 hours in the hospital. Pediatric patients need follow-up care after serious accidents. A patient of any age may need chemotherapy, physical therapy, or other kinds of help. Diabetic management can be done with home care. Many home care patients are elderly. Hospice patients may be included.

Nurses are widely employed in home health care, and many more will be needed in the future. Home health care is discussed in more detail in Unit 5.

UNIT 4/EXPANDED SETTINGS FOR HEALTH CARE DELIVERY 61

FACTORS INFLUENCING THE CHOICE OF CARE SETTING

One of the most important factors in choosing health care is money. The very wealthy may hire personal private duty nurses to live in their homes and give care. Those with limited income will often do without health care until they are acutely ill and require hospitalization. The rest of the population will choose care according to what their insurance company or family budget will allow. When personal resources are depleted and insurance benefits are gone, Medicaid (government monies) will be needed.

Another factor in choosing health care is availability. Some areas of the country have more choices to offer than others. People in larger cities often have access to several types of facilities. Residents of less populated areas will have fewer choices or have to travel greater distances for the kind of care they want.

The need for health care is a factor, too. A dull ache may not interfere with most daily activities and may be ignored. A sudden problem will force the person to seek help, sometimes without regard for costs. Age and sociocultural factors also influence the kind of care sought.

Knowledge of various kinds of care is another factor to consider. Many people remain unaware of the facilities available even in their own communities until a crisis arises in their life. Public education remains a very important goal of all health care services.

Along with knowledge, people must have a certain degree of trust in the health care system before they will seek help. In some cultures, folk medicine and home remedies are common practice; for many, doctors and nurses remain a last resort.

✳ KEY CONCEPT: FACTORS IN MAKING HEALTH CARE CHOICES

- Budget
- Availability
- Need
- Knowledge
- Trust

SUMMARY

Many changes are seen in the way health care is delivered in traditional settings. Hospitalized patients are acutely ill and are discharged earlier than ever before. Technology has further complicated patient care. Pediatric patients are no longer hospitalized unless they are critically ill. Parents must be taught caregiving skills for use at home. More pediatric care is now done in offices and clinics. In figure 4–6, a child is being examined for otitis media.

New settings are rapidly being developed. Ambulatory surgery centers, specialized types of day care centers, hospices, and community homes are just some examples. Home health care is another area where rapid growth of services is seen. Many of these settings will provide additional employment opportunities for nurses.

Nurses who are generalists will be adaptable in many care settings. You may be able to assist in the development of additional new settings in the future.

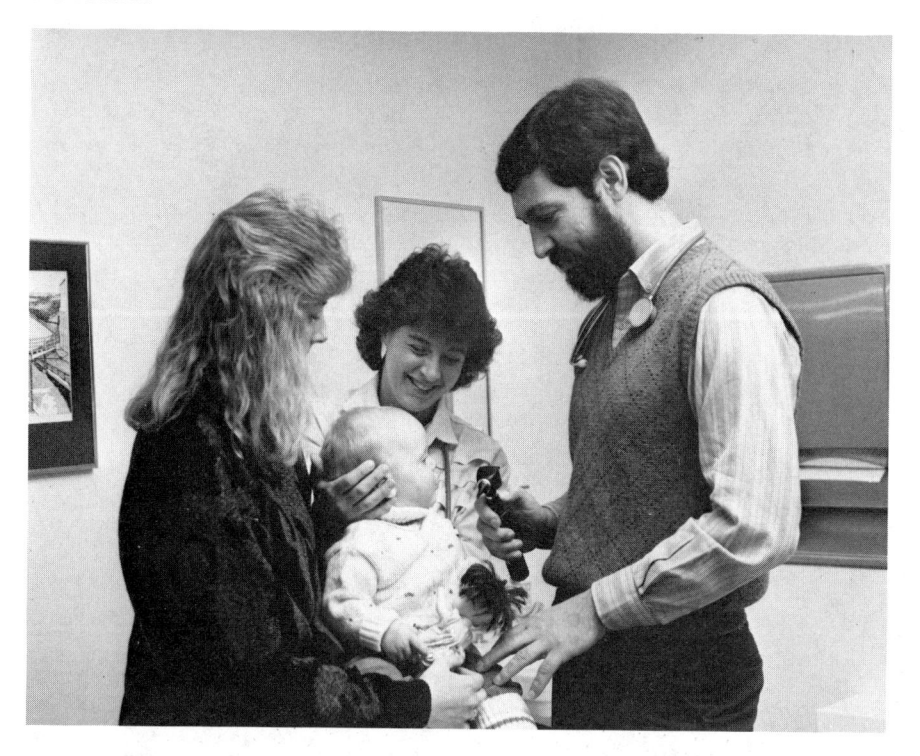

Figure 4–6 More pediatric care is now done in offices and clinics.

FOR DISCUSSION

- What kinds of expanded health care settings exist in your community? What are the roles of the nurses they employ?

- What kinds of expanded health care settings are needed in your community? Is there a need that you could help fill?

- How can health care workers increase the public knowledge and trust in existing settings?

QUESTIONS FOR REVIEW

1. List three ways nursing roles have changed in traditional care settings.
2. What is meant by "expanded settings" for health care?
3. List four expanded settings that employ nurses.
4. Identify four factors that influence the patient's choice of care setting.
5. Define *autonomy*. Give an example of a nurse making an autonomous decision.

5

Home Health Care: A Returning Alternative

OBJECTIVES:

After completing this unit, you will be able to:

- Distinguish between home health care and home care.
- Explain three types of home health care programs.
- Discuss the major reasons for the return to home health care.
- Discuss the roles of nurses in home health care agencies.
- Explain how a home health care agency works.

A large percentage of people in this country received medical care in their homes well into the mid-1900s or until doctors stopped making house calls. This unit will explain how health care has made a full circle in returning patients to their homes, or leaving them in their homes, for much of their treatment and subsequent recovery or death.

The development of the present home health care industry will be discussed. Three main types of home health care programs will be reviewed: public agencies, proprietory programs, and hospital–based programs. The process of arranging home health care will be reviewed, and several roles of nurses in home health care will be explained.

A distinction must be made between *home care* and *home health care*. Home health care includes those services given by nurses and nursing assistants to the ill or disabled person, figure 5–1. It also includes the specific health services of other health professionals, such as physical therapist, nutritionist, and physician. The health care of the patient is usually coordinated by the physician or nurse, and the patient.

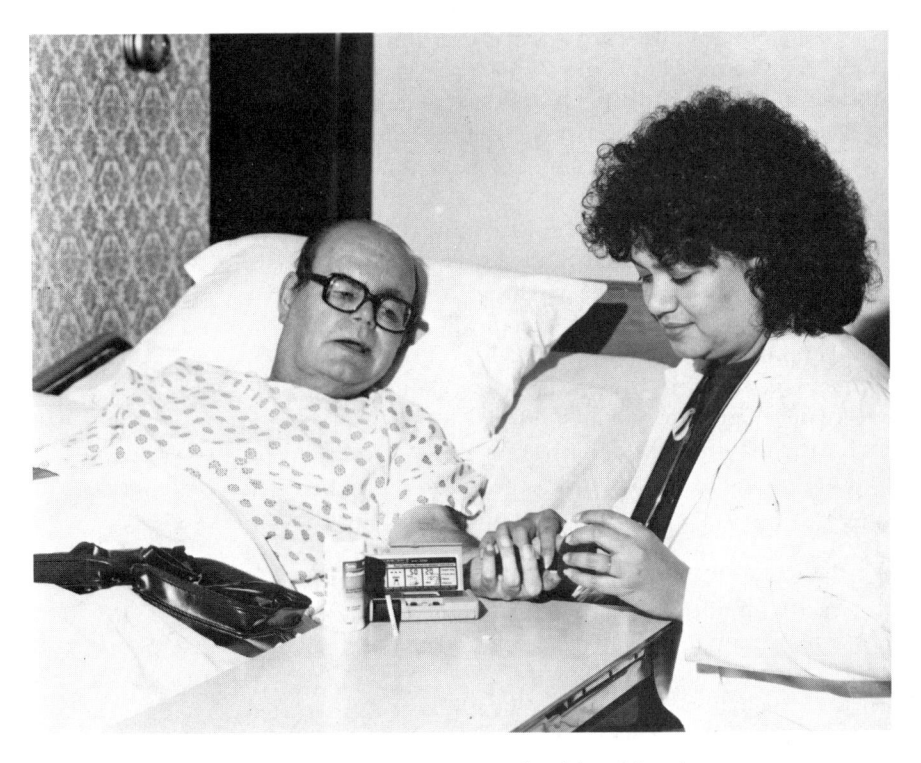

Figure 5–1 Home health nurse checking blood sugar

Home care, however, while it includes some basic personal care of the person's needs, such as bathing, is also designed to assist with other household tasks such as laundry, meal preparation, and light housekeeping. Sometimes homemaker aides are employed to provide these kinds of services. Transportation, shopping, and chore services may also be included. This care is often coordinated by a nurse or a social worker.

HISTORICAL REVIEW

Home health care issues have been documented for periods as early as 1796. Hospitals were considered pest houses where only the poor and indigent were sent. Most health care was given at home. It was generally accepted that patients were happier and had a better chance of recovery when they were treated at home.

The first government home health care service was initiated in Los Angeles County in 1898. The county hired nurses to teach cleanliness and home care skills to the ill and their families. Graduates of the first schools for practical nursing were expected to work in the homes of persons who were ill; the nurses were taught cooking and homemaking skills as well as how to give basic nursing care.

As hospitals became more numerous in the 1940s and 1950s, patients were often kept there for the duration of their illnesses. In addition, urbanization and mobility combined to break up the extended family. Technology aided in the growth of institutionalizing health care until separation of the ill from the family and community became the norm.

People had a tremendous belief in the power of medicine and science. Specialized facilities were developed for special kinds of problems. Hospitals were built for the care of the mentally ill. Sanatoriums were established for patients with tuberculosis. Nursing homes for the care of the dependent elderly followed the passage of the Medicare provisions under Social Security in 1965.

Private duty nurses have always been available for home care of the ill or disabled. These nurses are hired by the patient or family as independent contractors. They work independently of any agency and make their own payment arrangements with the patient.

Figure 5–2 illustrates the historical cycling of health care as it related to birthing. Today even those newborns who are born in hospitals may be sent home after 24 hours. Many HMOs contract with a home health nurse to make a home visit for teaching, assessment, and to obtain a blood sample for PKU (phenylketonuria) testing.

HOME HEALTH CARE TODAY

Home health care is part of comprehensive, total health care, as defined in figure 5–3. Home health care promotes, maintains, or restores health. It should help a person remain as independent as possible during chronic or terminal illness. It should help a person be independent in spite of some disability. Home health care should be individualized to the patient's needs.

Reasons for Development

There are several reasons for the re-emergence of home health care. The first is the consumers' demand to have the right to make their own decisions on health matters. This is partly in response to their perception that services are depersonalized, particularly in large institutions. Consumers insist on

Before 1900	Most births occur at home.
1920	95 percent of births occur at home. The use of forceps and episiotomy began in hospitals. Hospital births are promoted as safer.
1936	75 percent of births occur in hospitals. General anesthesia is common practice.
1950s–1960s	95 percent of births occur in hospitals. Hospital maternity services were organized like assembly lines. Women's movement beginning.
1970s	Books opposing births in hospitals are published. Alternate Birthing Centers (ABC) open in Connecticut, New York, New Mexico, California.
1976	Obstetricians oppose home births. Nurse midwife programs are expanding.
1980s	Birthing rooms are included in many hospital maternity units. Nurse midwives receive approval for payment from third-party payers. Number of home births is increasing.

Figure 5–2 History of birthing in the United States (Adapted from *Home Healthcare* by Allen D. Spiegel by permission of the publisher. Copyright 1983 by National Health Publishing Ltd. Partnership)

Home health care is that component of a continuum of comprehensive health care whereby services are provided to individuals and families in their places of residence for the purpose of promoting, maintaining, or restoring health or maximizing the level of independence while minimizing the effects of disability and illness including terminal illness. Services appropriate to the needs of the individual patient and family are planned, coordinated and made available by providers organized for the delivery of home health care through the use of employed staff, contractual arrangements, or a combination of the two patterns.

Figure 5–3 Definition of home health care (Adapted from *Home Healthcare* by Allen D. Spiegel by permission of the publisher. Copyright 1983 by National Health Publishing Ltd. Partnership)

receiving quality care with the personal touch. Sometimes patients feel as if they are strangers, intruders, or foreigners to the system that exists in hospitals.

Patients in home health care, however, remain the masters of their destiny. The health professionals who come into the home are guests there; the patient remains in control. Some authorities claim that this is why many people recover more rapidly in their own homes.

The second reason for the current increase in home health care is the economy. As the costs of health care escalated, many factors interacted to create a resurrection of home health care as a major focus. Because technology is so expensive, institutional health care has become a luxury item for all but the critically ill. Many researchers claim that quality health care can be delivered at home for much less cost.

A third factor in the growth of home health care is technology. With the miniaturization of computers and other high tech machinery, much can be done in the home as well as it is done in the hospital. Once patients and families become accustomed to the particular technology involved, they can manage quite well at home. Sometimes the home health nurse's primary role is that of teacher and trouble-shooter.

Examples of high tech home health care possibilities include: hyperalimentation, cancer chemotherapy via IV or implanted pump, intravenous antibiotic therapy, diabetic therapy with an insulin pump, home dialysis, tracheostomy ventilator care.

KEY CONCEPT: OVERVIEW OF HOME HEALTH CARE

- In the past health care was given in the home.
- Reasons for increasing home health care are:
    1) the patient is in control.
    2) it is less expensive than hospital care.
    3) technology can be adapted to the home use.
- Home health nurses are guests in the patient's home.

Philosophy of Home Health Care

The primary concept of home health care is that the patient truly is the center of the care provided. The patient and the family control the care;

all receive strength from being in their own environment. They do not have to adjust to schedules arranged by others. They do not have to limit visitors unless they want to.

Sometimes home health care nurses need to be reminded that in the home setting, the nurse is the guest. The patient may choose the time and duration of care and has the right to refuse care. The home health care nurse is not intended to be the primary caregiver; he or she is to assist, support, and educate the family member who has taken that role.

TYPES OF HOME HEALTH CARE PROGRAMS

Public Health Agencies

Throughout the twentieth century community health nurses have been employed by county and state health departments to provide basic health care to citizens. These agencies receive government funding for their operation. Many of their programs are focused on certain categories, such as mothers and newborn infants, young children, and low-income families. Most public agencies provide health screening services and educational information.

Consumers of public health services are expected to contribute to the cost of their care according to their ability to pay. Most public health home care agencies are approved for funding by Medicare/Medicaid.

Public health nurses (PHN) are registered nurses (RNs) with degrees in public health. The director of a public agency is usually a public health nurse. Other registered nurses, licensed practical/vocational nurses (LP/VNs), and home health aides may be employed by these agencies.

Proprietary Agencies

Proprietary agencies are businesses that are organized to make a profit. At the present time, Upjohn Health Care Service, Inc., is reported to be the largest proprietary agency; in 1969 they had 37 offices across the country; in 1980 they had expanded to 260 offices. The growth of private companies in this area of service is rapid. An agency started by a doctor in 1974, Quality Care, Inc., began with five offices; in 1981 that agency had 180 offices in 45 states.

Customers of proprietary agencies are charged fees according to the level of care needed. Skilled nursing services, provided by an RN or an LP/VN, are more costly than services given by a home health aide. Some proprietary agencies have applied for and been given approval for Medicare or Medicaid funding. Many traditional health insurance plans do not cover home health care yet, although some HMOs do.

These agencies must have an RN or a physician as a consultant in order to qualify for Medicare/Medicaid funding. Other RNs, LP/VNs, and home health aides are employed by proprietary groups. Some proprietors also employ or contract with other health care providers such as occupational therapists and social workers.

Hospital-Based Programs

The newest entry into home health care are those programs operated by acute care hospitals. Many hospitals are developing home health care units as a way of extending their services. Ideally, the home health nurses can be involved in the hospital discharge planning process, and coordination of care should be quite smooth.

Paying for home health care through a hospital-based program involves the same alternatives as through a proprietary agency. These programs may also apply for certification for Medicare and Medicaid patients.

The home health nurses in hospital-based programs are employees of the hospital. In some situations, they may work part time in the acute care unit and part time in the home health unit. RNs, LP/VNs and home health aides may be included.

Regulation of Home Health Care Agencies

Because of the recent and rapid growth of all types of home health services, there is not yet much regulation. States vary in how agencies may qualify for certification. Some states have established only minimal licensing requirements.

Medicare and Medicaid regulations are the primary source of government control of home health care at this time. In order to be Medicare certified, the agency must have written care plans and send a written report to the doctor every 60 days. They also must have an RN make the initial assessment, see the patient at least every two weeks, and train and supervise the home health aides. *Certification* means that the agency meets required standards established by the certifying group.

Agencies may also seek accreditation by a national group. *Accreditation* is voluntary, and it means the agency meets criteria established by the national group. The criteria are more than minimum requirements and accredited agencies are considered above average. The National League for Nursing (NLN) accredits those home health agencies that are not part of a hospital. The Joint Commission on Accreditation of Hospitals (JCAH) accredits hospital-based agencies. The National HomeCaring Council (NHC) and the Council on Accreditation of Services for Families and Children (COA) also accredit home health services.

The opportunity for fraud exists when any industry grows rapidly. Patients who seek home health care should be informed that not all advertised agencies may be qualified to give the type of care they need. Nurses who seek employment in home health care should also be aware that there are many differences between agencies.

KEY CONCEPT: HOME HEALTH CARE PROGRAMS

Home health care services may be provided by:

- Public health agencies
- Proprietary agencies
- Hospital-based programs

Regulation of the industry is not uniform:

- Some states require licenses.
- Some agencies are Medicare certified.
- Agencies can seek accreditation.

HOW A HOME HEALTH CARE AGENCY WORKS

A home health care agency may learn of potential patients in several ways. The patient or a family member may contact an agency directly. Sometimes a neighbor may inquire, or the patient's clergy may make the initial contact. This may be in response to advertisement or through word-of-mouth publicity. A physician may refer a patient to the agency. A hospital nurse or social worker may contact the agency about a patient who needs help after hospital discharge, figure 5–4.

The agency's case coordinator, usually a PHN, then makes arrangements to visit the patient. This may be done while the patient is still hospitalized or at home. The coordinator will usually contact the physician for

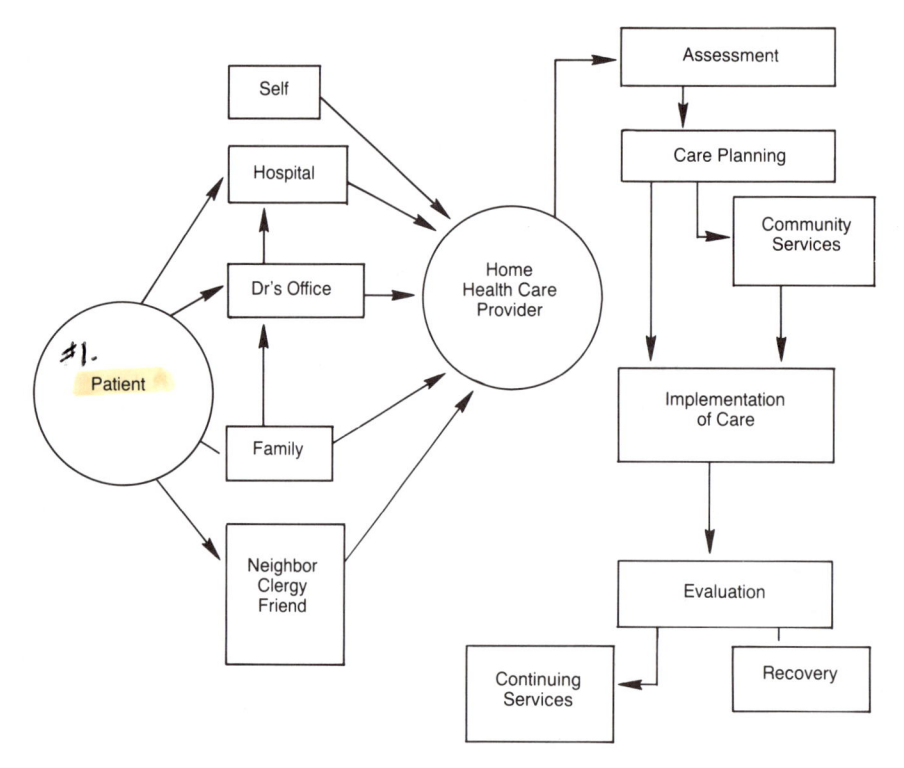

Figure 5-4 Patient movement through home care agency

specific orders about medications or treatments. The initial assessment interview will enable the case coordinator to decide whether or not home health care is needed. Payment arrangements will also be reviewed, because the kind of services allowed will make a difference in care planning. A sample assessment tool useful for the first home health care visit can be found in Appendix B.

Care Planning

Once the decision for home health care is made, the next decision is what kind of help is needed. This will be based on the patient's specific needs and the doctor's instructions. The wishes of the family must also be considered. The care plan must include the kind of nursing care to be given and the number of hours of care required.

If the home needs modification for care of the patient, it should be arranged before the patient comes home. Perhaps special equipment will be needed, such as a hospital bed, commode, or walker. If high tech equipment will be used, the home should be assessed for adequate electrical outlets and a back-up generator should be obtained.

Case Assignment

If the patient will need intermittent skilled nursing care for a specific treatment, an RN or LP/VN may be assigned to the case. *Intermittent* means at intervals; for example, the nurse might visit the patient once daily for two weeks. Perhaps this could be to supervise insulin administration and continue diabetic education.

A nurse could also be assigned to draw a blood specimen for coagulation studies when a patient is receiving heparin therapy at home, figure 5–5. The nurse will also be expected to make many observations as well as carry out specific treatments that require nursing knowledge. Sterile dressing changes, administration of intravenous antibiotics, emotional support, and patient teaching are other examples.

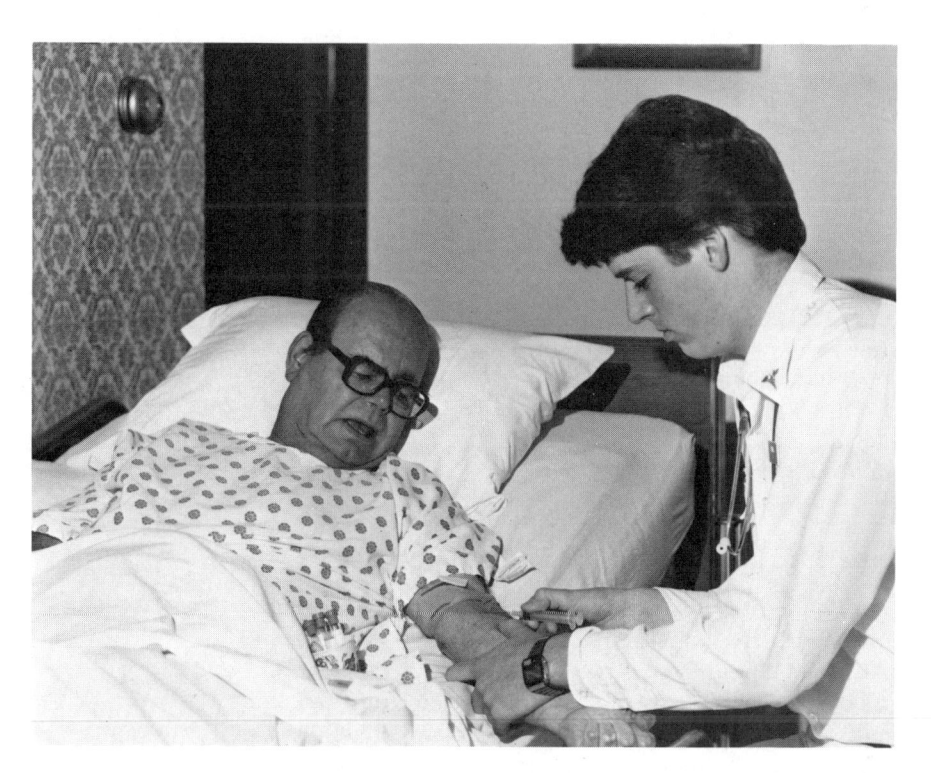

Figure 5–5 Home health nurse completing a venipuncture

Occasionally a patient needs constant skilled nursing care. Then several qualified nurses will be assigned. An example of this situation would be a patient with a tracheostomy who is on a ventilator.

Sometimes a patient needs help only with bathing and dressing. These duties may be assigned to a home health aide. A nurse will visit all patients served by the agency on a regular basis to determine if the patient's needs are being met effectively.

Other kinds of health care workers may also be involved with a particular patient. Some agencies employ or have contracts with physical therapists, speech therapists, and psychologists. Type of payment may influence the case assignment. Medicare and some other third party payers specify the hours and caregivers that will be covered.

Care Conferences

The case coordinator will hold a weekly care conference about every patient. Sometimes these meetings may be conducted by telephone. The nurses and aides caring for that patient should participate, as well as any special health workers involved in that patient's case. In some situations, the patient or a family member may also attend the conference. As with hospital care conferences, this meeting should be used to plan and to evaluate the care given.

The hospice patient in home health care is in a very special situation. The entire hospice team should be involved in regular conferences for continuity of patient care and as part of the overall support system.

Recordkeeping

Home health agencies must keep thorough records. The nurses, aides, and other workers have notes to add to the record. Many times third party payers require documentation before they will pay for the services. Recordkeeping includes employee records as well as patients' charts.

Terminating Home Health Care

Some home health care patients will continue to need assistance for many years. Others will only need nurses for a relatively short time. It is important for the case coordinator and the nurses to recognize when the patient and family are able to take over. If the care was primarily for education, for example, then it would be a short-term arrangement, as anticipated from the beginning.

> **KEY CONCEPT: OPERATION OF A HOME HEALTH CARE AGENCY**
>
> - Referral leads to an initial assessment.
> - Care planning is done with the patient.
> - Assignments depend on patient's needs and the payment plan.
> - Care conferences are held weekly.
> - Thorough records are kept.
> - Services may be temporary or long term.

SUMMARY

The home health care industry has grown rapidly due to cost containment efforts in hospitals and due to patients' desires to be in command. Even complicated care can be managed at home with new technologies, competent nurses, and willing families.

Home health care agencies may be public, proprietary or hospital-based. Payment for home health care varies. There is not yet much regulation of the home health care industry.

Patients may be referred for home health care by any interested person, including themselves. A PHN should coordinate the care, assigning nurses and aides according to the patient's needs. Other health workers may also be involved in home health care.

FOR DISCUSSION

- What kinds of home health care agencies are available in your community? What kinds of services will they provide? What types of nurses do they employ?
- Do you think quality health care can be given at home? What kinds of patients would benefit most from home health care?
- What are some qualities needed by the home health nurse? Do you think you would enjoy being a nurse in someone's home?

- Consider some of the patients you have met in your clinical experiences to date. Are there any who could have been cared for at home?

QUESTIONS FOR REVIEW

1. Explain the difference between home health care and home care.
2. Identify two reasons for the growth in home health care.
3. What is the difference between a public health agency and a proprietary home health care agency?
4. What kinds of things does a nurse generalist do in home health care?
5. How does someone become a home health care patient?

SECTION TWO

COMMUNITIES' RESPONSIBILITY FOR HEALTH CARE

Unit 6 Communities and Their Health

Unit 7 The Team Concept of Community and Home Care

Unit 8 Community and Home Care Team Members

Section Two builds on the nurse's knowledge of the health care delivery system. It is designed to stretch the boundaries of the nursing team and health care team. These groups have been viewed as clusters of health professionals and caregivers in a health care facility; they have been the operating room (OR) team, the cardiac team, Team One on Station 3–C, or the medical–surgical nurses.

The expanded settings of health care delivery moves the health care team out into the community and includes additional services that are indirectly involved in a patient's health.

This section guides the nurse in identifying population groups with health risks. The roles of known caregivers are adapted to new settings, and new members added to the community health team. The section concludes with a review of cultural influences that will assist the nurse in practicing health care in expanded settings.

6

Communities and Their Health

OBJECTIVES:

After completing this unit, you will be able to:

- Define communities by groups of people with specific health concerns.
- Identify a specific community group and its specific health concerns.
- Discuss public and private agencies that are involved in identifying and meeting health needs of a community.
- Discuss the role of the nurse in promoting health in a variety of community groups.

This unit will guide you in beginning to view the United States, and the world, as a large community. Within this community are hundreds of smaller communities made up of specialized groups with specific health concerns. The members of these groups may be identified by their work, where they live, their ethnic origin, or other mutual bonds.

There are many public and private agencies that are watch dogs in keeping areas of our environment as safe as possible to promote health and prevent disease. *Watch dogs* are groups of people that are alert to activities, or watch them, in order to prevent waste or unethical practices. The Environmental Protection Agency (EPA) is an example of such a public agency. There are also consumer interest groups that observe for signs of problems. Nurses should be active members of this group. They are often the grass-roots observers of specific concerns such as identifying the need for explaining special diets to the elderly or immunizing preschoolers in a depressed community.

UNIT 6/COMMUNITIES AND THEIR HEALTH

This unit will present examples of specific community groups and their health concerns, agencies that assist with the concerns, and how nurses fit in this process.

DEFINING COMMUNITIES

In the past doctors and nurses as well as other caregivers focused on the needs of persons in the community in which they lived. Today, with the rapid growth of technology in all areas of our lives, health concerns of people in other countries affect the health of our own community. As the flu season strikes each year we hear about the "Hong Kong flu" or the "Asian flu." Newspapers describe how these viruses travel from continent to continent. In the spring of 1986 the Soviet Union's Chernobyl nuclear plant accident raised health concern issues worldwide.

People are more mobile as they travel from state to state and country to country. You have probably read about a restaurant that has closed temporarily due to customers becoming ill with hepatitis. It is often a challenge for the health department to locate the customers at risk because they may live hundreds of miles away from the restaurant. The community identified here would be the customers of a specific restaurant.

In 1976 the American Legion was identified as a community with a specific health concern. While at a convention in Philadelphia, 182 members became ill with a strange respiratory ailment. Twenty-nine Legionnaires died. Their plight became known as Legionnaires' Disease.

Other community groups with health concerns have included young women who used some brands of tampons during menstruation. They were at risk to develop Toxic Shock Syndrome. Another community at risk in the 1980s is the children who are given aspirin for treatment of influenza. They may have their illness complicated by Reye's Syndrome. Most recently, the gay community was identified to be at risk to contract AIDS (acquired immune deficiency syndrome).

LOOKING AT WORLD-WIDE HEALTH CONCERNS

As technology has made our world smaller, we have world current events at our fingertips via satellite. The famine in Africa was made an international concern in the summer of 1985 with the "Live Aid" concert. A record called "We are the World" was made to raise funds for thousands of starving people. This was not the first time the eyes of the world have focused on

Africa's nutrition problem. Recurring droughts and limited knowledge about agricultural technology have been responsible for nutritional deficiencies over the years.

In Japan the diet of fish and fresh vegetables results in a low incidence of cholesterol-related diseases and rectal cancer. However, the high sodium content of seasonings in the diet may lead to problems such as hypertension.

In the United States the number one cause of death is heart disease. This condition is directly related to lifestyle choices. A diet high in salt and saturated fats, lack of exercise, and increased stress are all contributing factors.

During this century the medical community, government regulatory agencies, nurses, and many others have had to change the focus of research, laws, and caregiving. At the turn of the century most of the deaths of three large communities (men, women, and children) were related to infections. The leading cause of death for men was tuberculosis; women, pneumonia; and children, diarrhea. The influenza epidemic of 1918 killed millions of people—not just in the United States, but worldwide.

Today lifestyle-related conditions claim the majority of lives in the United States. In addition to cardiovascular diseases, lung cancer is increasing in women, and more children die from accidents than any other cause.

KEY CONCEPT: SAMPLES OF WORLD HEALTH CONCERNS

- Nutrition-related problems such as famine afflict third world countries.
- Lifestyle-related problems such as decreased exercise and increased stress lead to cardiovascular disorders.
- Problems, such as AIDS, are related to social behavior.

LOOKING AT U.S. HEALTH CONCERNS

To identify specific communities with specific health concerns, the United States can be divided many times geographically. These divisions include regional areas with several states, rural areas, and urban areas. Even within these urban areas, neighborhoods may have different health concerns.

The rural community may have cleaner air and fresher farm produce but have concerns with contaminated ground water because of using pesticides in fields. The people may not have quick access to medical care. The general urban area may have high tech medical care within minutes of their home, but are at risk with air and water pollution from industrial sites.

A concern of inner city neighborhoods is often housing. There are many homeless, as the limited housing is often unaffordable and frequently substandard. A community within this neighborhood is the mentally handicapped group. Because of the closing of many state and mental hospitals, this population has been integrated into the community. However, comprehensive social services have not been able to meet the needs of these persons. Many have drifted to the inner city and become street people or single room occupants (SROs) of inexpensive hotels or rooming houses.

Neighborhood communities may be defined as apartments for single persons, elderly high-rises, or mobile home parks. Communities with elderly persons will have concerns regarding transportation, nutrition programs, and safety in housing, Figure 6–1. Builders of housing for the elderly are becoming more aware of the need for handrails in bathrooms, signals to an office, and non-glare lighting. Federally subsidized housing for the elderly and handicapped now must follow safety regulations. This includes mailboxes inside the building, light switches placed lower on the walls, and wider doorways to accommodate wheelchairs. As the general population grows older, perhaps we will see larger numbers and letters on thermostats, stoves, and water faucets.

KEY CONCEPT: SAMPLES OF U.S. HEALTH CONCERNS

- Rural—lack of immediate accessible health care
- Urban—threats from industrial pollution and concerns because of inadequate housing
- Neighborhoods—transportation and nutrition concerns for specific groups such as the elderly

---

ADDITIONAL COMMUNITIES IDENTIFIED

Ethnic Communities

Ethnic communities in the United States have identified specific health risks and concerns. Examples include the native American, black American, Hispanic, and Asian immigrant communities.

Clinics in native American neighborhoods provide care and health education for identified health risks of diabetes, hypertension, obesity, and alcoholism. The high infant mortality rate in the native American population has led to the aggressive development of prenatal programs.

Sickle-cell anemia consulting clinics for blacks are available. Hypertension, diabetes, and obesity are among other conditions prevalent among blacks.

Health risks identified in the Hispanic community are those identified largely with below-average family incomes. These conditions include obesity, diabetes, hypertension, and respiratory and gastrointestinal conditions.

During the 1970s and early 1980s many Asian immigrants came to the United States from refugee camps. Conditions such as tuberculosis, intestinal parasites, and malnutrition were evident. The immigrants also needed emotional help with adjustments to the American culture.

Work-Related Communities

Communities can include groups with similar jobs and professions. Each level of worker within the industry can be regrouped into other communities. Factory line workers may be at risk for accidents with machinery. Upper management workers may be at risk for stress-related cardiovascular diseases. With the movement toward preventing illness, many industries are implementing wellness programs.

Asbestosis is a work-related disease. The community at risk are workers in industries where asbestos fibers can be inhaled. Examples are the construction industry—where the asbestos is used in a prefabricated form—and the fireproofing and textile industries. Asbestos is also used in the manufacture of automobile brake and clutch linings.

Coal miners are at risk to develop Black Lung Disease. This is caused by inhalation and prolonged retention of coal dust particles.

The Federal Occupation Safety and Health Act (OSHA) protects against potential hazards of the workplace. In some occupations, workers are now required to wear surgical masks, steel-toed shoes, or other protective clothing. Individual states are involved in developing safety awareness in employees, figure 6–2.

School Communities

Schools include a variety of communities. Age-related concerns can be identified. The neighborhood where the school is located and the socioeconomic level of the students' parents are contributing factors. Latch Key children have been identified with the increasing number of working mothers. These children may wear, on a chain around their necks, the key to the family

UNIT 6/COMMUNITIES AND THEIR HEALTH 83

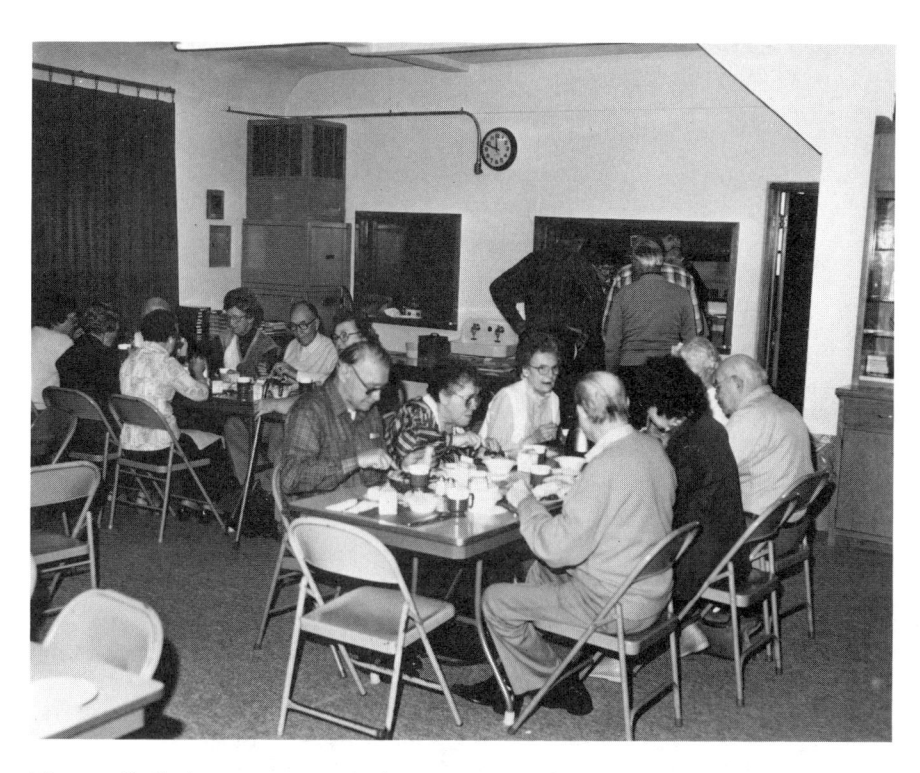

Figure 6–1 A target population group: senior citizens' nutritional needs are met through congregate dining.

home. They are home alone after school until a parent returns from work. Safety is obviously a key issue for them.

Nutrition programs in schools have been in effect for many years. Children who would otherwise start their school day on an empty stomach may receive breakfast at their school. Hot lunch programs have been implemented for decades.

College campuses provide another school community. Students arrive from many areas, states, countries, and have different value systems. They develop new bonds and needs within their new community. The stress of preparing for life goals and developing independence are often predisposing factors in compromising the body's immune system. Childhood communicable diseases have emerged as a campus community threat, figure 6–3. Immunizations have protected the public for decades; unfortunately, some parents are no longer alert to the need to follow infant immunization programs.

Each person may be a member of many health concern groups. Membership may change when he or she changes jobs, takes a vacation, or joins a special interest group.

> ### KEY CONCEPT: SOME SPECIFIC COMMUNITIES' HEALTH CONCERNS
>
> - Ethnic communities
>   - Native Americans—high infant mortality rate
>   - Blacks—sickle-cell anemia and hypertension
>   - Hispanics—conditions seen in low-income populations
>   - Asian Refugees—cultural adjustments
> - Work-related communities
>   - Factory line workers—machinery accidents
>   - Management workers—stress-related conditions
> - School communities
>   - Lower socioeconomic level—nutrition concerns
>   - College students—new outbreak of measles
> - People belong to many communities at the same time

COMMUNITY INVOLVEMENT IN HEALTH CONCERNS

In the previous section, the history of the health care delivery system and the developing changes that occurred were examined. The focus on social change and desire for a better living and working environment have promoted and sometimes provoked laws, regulations, and the formation of watch dog agencies.

Today the government is involved at the federal, state, and local level in responding to the health concerns and risks of many target populations. A *target population* may be defined as an isolated group of people with an identified specific health concern. They may be isolated with respect to age, geography, ethnicity, workplace, or other mutual identities.

The Federal Government has environmental regulations to protect the air we breathe and the water we drink. There are also funds for programs

MINNESOTA
"EMPLOYEE RIGHT TO KNOW ACT OF 1983"

INTRODUCTION

The Employee Right-to-Know Act was passed by the State Legislature during the 1983 session and revised in both the 1984 and 1985 sessions. It is enforced as part of the Occupational Safety and Health program in the Department of Labor and Industry. This brochure briefly highlights the main points of the law. It is not intended to cover all of the technical aspects involved which are only available by reviewing the statute and the standards.

SUMMARY OF THE LAW

The Employee Right-To-Know Act is intended to ensure that employees are aware of the dangers associated with hazardous substances, harmful physical agents, or infectious agents (in hospitals and clinics) that they may be exposed to in their workplaces. The Act requires employers to evaluate their workplaces for the presence of hazardous substances, harmful physical agents, and infectious agents and to provide training to employees concerning those substances or agents to which employees may be exposed. Written information on hazardous substances, harmful physical agents or infectious agents must be readily accessible to employees or their representatives. Employees have a conditional right to refuse to work under imminent danger conditions. Labelling requirements for containers of hazardous substances and equipment or work areas that generate harmful physical agents are also included in the Act.

EMPLOYEE RIGHTS

- To receive information and training on "Hazardous Substances," "Harmful Physical Agents," or "Infectious Agents" to which they may be exposed.
- To be trained on the hazards of the above prior to initial assignment to work with the substance or agent and to receive a yearly training update.
- To refuse to work under imminent danger conditions.

EMPLOYER RIGHTS

- To assign employees to alternative jobs until hazardous conditions can be eliminated.
- To request a signed statement from employees verifying that training was received.
- Protection of trade secrets.

INFECTIOUS AGENTS

Hospitals and clinics must provide training to their employees on infectious agents to which those employees are routinely exposed. The training program must include the chain of infection, techniques to avoid self-contamination, hazards to special at-risk groups, recommended immunization practices, and how to obtain additional information.

Figure 6-2 Employee Right to Know Act (Courtesy of the Minnesota Department of Labor and Industry)

to meet specific needs of smaller target groups. Through the Older Americans Act, the Meals-on-Wheels program provides one hot meal five days a week, delivered to shut-ins. A similar program called *congregate dining* provides a meal in a central location to people over 60 years of age.

Each state has its own guidelines for licensing health care facilities and persons providing the care. State health departments inspect and monitor restaurants for compliance with regulations. Agencies, including the census bureau, gather data from birth to death in order to identify risks, concerns, and trends. Based on this data, the population of persons over 65 will double during the last quarter of this century. By the twenty-first century, 20 percent of the people in the United States will be over 65; this population is the greatest user of health care services.

Each community has sanitation plants and waste removal services to protect the local environment. Federal as well as local funds are used to

GUSTAVUS ADOLPHUS COLLEGE

Saint Peter, Minnesota 56082
Telephone (507) 931-8000

August 21, 1985

Dear Gustie:

Since January 15 of this year there have been several outbreaks of Measles (Rubeola) and German Measles (Rubella) on college campuses. Measles outbreaks have occurred at the Ohio State University, Boston University and Principia College in Elsah, Illinois.

Because college-age students are at high risk for contracting these diseases, and because of the potential seriousness of a campus outbreak, we urge you to take the following steps BEFORE you return to campus in the fall:

1. REVIEW YOUR IMMUNIZATION RECORDS.

2. IF YOU ARE IMMUNE TO MEASLES AND RUBELLA, VERIFY YOUR IMMUNITY BY COMPLETING THE ENCLOSED SHEET. SEND OR BRING THE SHEET TO THE HEALTH SERVICE, GUSTAVUS ADOLPHUS COLLEGE, ST. PETER, MN 56082.

3. IF YOU ARE NOT IMMUNE, GET THE APPROPRIATE VACCINATION(S) AND SEND OR BRING THE ENCLOSED SHEET TO THE HEALTH SERVICE.

   Acceptable proof of immunization consists of:

   a) A personal or parental written record which includes the month and year of immunization, or

   b) A written record from a high school or college previously attended, or

   c) A record from a physician or a public immunization clinic.

Once again, we URGE you to take care of this matter BEFORE you return for fall semester. We hope you are and will continue to enjoy the summer. Thank you.

Sincerely yours,

Mary Jean Richter, Head Nurse
Gustavus Health Service

Bruce A. Gray
Dean of Students

mm
encl.

Figure 6–3 Current health concerns in the college community (Courtesy of Gustavus Adolphus College, St. Peter, Minnesota)

> ## KEY CONCEPT: AGENCIES ADDRESSING HEALTH CONCERNS
>
> - Federal Government provides funds for target populations such as programs for the elderly through the Older Americans Act.
> - State Governments license health care agencies and personnel.
> - Local Governments utilize funds from all government levels, provide sanitation services, and implement nutrition, transportation, and other services.
> - Private Agencies and Volunteer Groups collect funds and provide services and education to target groups.
> - Consumer Advocates collect information related to consumer concerns and bring them to the attention of the general public and the lawmakers.

provide and improve services through community government, the schools, and interested citizen groups.

Additional agencies include private and volunteer groups. Usually these groups have a single interest focus; examples are the American Heart Association, Diabetes Association, and the Association for Alzheimer's and Related Diseases. For many years entertainer Jerry Lewis has raised millions of dollars during the Labor Day telethon for the Muscular Dystrophy Association. The American Red Cross provides a variety of services and volunteers on the international level.

The purpose of the many private and volunteer groups is to provide education and support to those affected with a specific condition. They also educate the general public, direct the fundraising, and promote research.

Community involvement in health-related issues has been influenced considerably by special interest groups and social reform. There was much social unrest in the United States in the 1960s. President Lyndon Johnson's "Great Society" gave birth to a wide variety of social programs. The Civil Rights Act of 1964 opened the door for opportunities and services for minority populations. The neglected health care of the elderly was identified. With the rapidly rising cost of health care, retired citizens with no health

Table 6-1 "Great Society" social programs

FOCUS OF GOVERNMENT	GOVERNMENT SPONSORED PROGRAMS

War on Poverty	Economic Opportunity Act, 1964
	Job Corps–Vocational training of disadvantaged youth
	Community Action Program
	  Project Head Start–for disadvantaged preschoolers
	Work Experience Program
	  child day care and other support programs
	VISTA (Volunteers in Service to America)–domestic Peace Corps volunteers work and teach in ghettos
	The Food Stamp Program assists low income families to stretch food dollars

End Racial Injustice	Civil Rights Acts 1964–barred discrimination in employment 1965–Voting Rights Act banned literacy tests 1968–barred discrimination in rental and sale of housing
Expansion of Social Welfare Programs	Social Security Act amended for Medicare and Medicaid
Environmental Protection	Water Quality Act of 1965 Clean Air Act of 1965 established auto emission standards

Consumerism	Fair Packaging and Labeling Act of 1966
	  content and net quantity listed on labels
	Wholesale Meat Act of 1967
	  all processing plants were subject to federal meat inspection

care insurance did not seek medical attention. In 1965 the Social Security Titles 18 and 19 were passed to assist the elderly with health care needs. These are more often known as Medicare and Medicaid. Many of the present changes in delivery of health care are a result of the unexpected accelerating cost of these programs. Table 6–1 identifies some social programs born in the 1960s.

Another influence that emerged in the social unrest of the 1960s was the consumer advocate. Ralph Nader became assertive and well known in speaking out for the rights of the consumer. He rallied to promote regulations for safer automobiles, identified consumer fraud, testified on conditions in nursing homes, and criticized inadequacies of government health and safety programs. (Refer to Key Concepts on page 87.)

IDENTIFYING AND RESOLVING COMMUNITY HEALTH RISKS

You are now able to place people in a number of groups where they have a mutual bond with other people with similar interests, concerns, and risks. Identifying health concerns or risks of a specific group can be a complex task.

One method of anticipating people at risk is through past experiences such as those resulting from natural disasters. Concerns about water contamination follow flooding. Meeting the basic needs of food, clothing, and shelter are problems which follow tornados, hurricanes, and other weather-related disasters.

Past experiences with social issues that present health risks include the previously discussed lifestyle of people with cardiovascular diseases. Crowded housing, when many people live in a small space, is known to produce increased incidence of disease such as tuberculosis.

Another method of identifying risks is looking more closely at technology. It has improved health care and rapid communication. On the other hand technology is often detrimental to our health. Industrial wastes that were of no concern a half century ago are priority concerns now. Acid rain affects the environment, crops, and food supplies. People with respiratory problems have to stay indoors during smog alerts. Contents of buried waste canisters leak into the underground water supply and contaminate drinking water. However, it is encouraging to learn that because of industrial waste control some lakes are cleaner than they were a decade ago.

How do these concerns become well known? Many times it is the people who work with or are involved with a specific group who identify the risk. It is the small-town doctor, the college health service, or the elementary school teacher who first identifies a new situation or observes a change that occurs in several people. This is the beginning of a risk or concern of a target population. Through existing channels (school nurse, state health department), the concern can be addressed and investigated. Frequent occurrences of a problem also increase the interest of researchers.

Research is also helped by the lobbying of special interest groups and political action. An example of this pressure in the late 1980s was the demand for preventive education and search for curative treatment for AIDS.

Research involves more than just identifying the community at risk or looking into a microscope. The community needs to be surveyed extensively. The health habits, lifestyle, industrial and environmental influences are only a few of the considerations in compiling data.

A plan for action to meet the potential or actual health risks of an identified group requires community awareness. There are many questions to ask. First, is the group aware of a potential or actual health risk? Secondly, are they willing to take action? A considerable amount of time and dollars can be spent on surveys, research, and planning, but if the target population does not cooperate, the effort will be in vain. An example refers to the popularity of fast-food restaurants. There has been considerable research and education to inform the public of the relationship between a diet high in sodium and unsaturated fats to the increase in cardiovascular diseases. Yet we still eat lots of hamburgers and french fries served by these restaurants.

The willingness to take action involves more groups than the community with the health risk. In many situations Federal Government health planning may be involved. Planning must consider the amount of money needed to meet the intended objective. Will this project require tax dollars and/or private donations? Time is another important factor. Is the risk an emergency situation or is it a long term, ongoing problem? An example, again, is the pressure on the government to research AIDS.

The anticipated difficulty in resolving the problem will also influence the willingness to take action on the problem. Will the target population comply? An example is smoking. Despite a warning on cigarette packages, smoking is increasing in some population groups.

The plan for action also considers the number of people involved and the cost of the plan in relation to the number of people that will benefit. Immunization programs are examples of plans that are cost effective and reach hundreds, often thousands of people. Politics and emotions, however, are involved in health care. Often what seems to be the logical chain of events does not occur. Serving the greatest number of people for the dollar seems reasonable but may not happen. The cost of maintaining life for one mechanical heart transplant patient would pay for the replacement of heart valves for 200 patients. One-third of all children in this country have never seen a dentist; the same monies could pay for their dental care. On the other hand, knowledge obtained from the research and experiences of the mechanical heart transplant could improve or maintain a quality of life for hundreds in the future.

KEY CONCEPT: METHODS OF IDENTIFYING HEALTH RISKS

- Past Experiences—natural disasters
- Effects of Technology—industrial wastes
- Increased Incidence of a Problem—overcrowded housing

KEY CONCEPT: METHODS OF RESOLVING HEALTH RISKS

- Research—stimulated by special interest groups and political action
- Community Awareness—prompted through the media and education
- Considerations for Action—time, money, consumer interest, and the number of people affected

---

NURSES IN THE COMMUNITY

Nurses are members of a geographical community as well as several health concern/risk target populations. They are grass roots observers of environmental and lifestyle influences. After completing a basic nursing program and beginning practice, they will be aware of health practices and potential health risks of the general population. In-service and continuing education programs help nurses to keep current with research and treatment trends. There are many nursing magazines today that assist the nurse in keeping up-to-date. Reading newspapers, news magazines, and following TV news and documentaries may provide nurses with the immediate health care issues and the response of the public.

As a health care provider, the nurse is a role model. The community looks to the nurse as a nonthreatening resource person. Do you recall beginning your basic nursing program? Friends, neighbors, and relatives were soon at your door seeking health advice!

Nurses need to be good resource persons and patient advocates in the community. By developing an alertness for information presented through local media, schools, churches, and other sources, the nurse acquires an extensive catalog of referral resources. The nurse should become aware of local meal services for the elderly, transportation services for senior citizens and the handicapped, free blood pressure check centers, and well-baby clinics. Providing a concerned neighbor with the correct information and telephone numbers makes the nurse a patient advocate and resource person.

Communities are becoming more responsive to the abused child and the vulnerable adult. States are passing laws addressing these concerns. Nurses have been identified as persons responsible to report observations indicating these abuses. Ethical and legal responsibilities will be detailed in the next section of this text.

Even when not on-the-job, nurses are resource persons. Consult the nurse practice act of your state to understand what is nursing practice and what is not; nurses do not practice medicine, they help resolve health problems.

KEY CONCEPT: NURSE'S COMMUNITY ROLE

- Be a Grass Roots observer of environmental and lifestyle influences on health.
- Keep up-to-date with current health care trends.
- Be a role model for good health habits.
- Be a resource person and advocate for patients.
- Practice within ethical and legal boundaries.

SUMMARY

This unit has presented a newer concept of health concerns. During basic nursing education you may have focused on the Intake and Output records of some hospitalized patients. You learned about their risk for postoperative problems or the complications of bedrest. Now you have knowledge about a variety of communities with mutual bonds and health concerns. You can view fluid intake needs in a new light: the starving populations of drought-stricken Africa or a community recovering from spring floods whose people cannot drink the contaminated water.

You have begun to learn about the influence of social change, concerned citizens, the media, politics, and costs on community health. As a nurse and citizen, you can place yourself in an expanded role of observer and reporter.

FOR DISCUSSION

- Identify three health risk communities in your area. Describe them and their health risks.
- Visit a health agency (federal, state, local, volunteer) and discuss their specific influence on area health.
- Interview a nurse who has been in practice several years. How does he/she view the role of the nurse as a referral person and patient advocate?

QUESTIONS FOR REVIEW

1. List four target population groups.
2. Identify two population groups and specific health risks of each group.
3. Identify one government agency and discuss how it meets the health needs of a community.
4. What legislation in the 1960s assisted in improving the health care for the elderly?
5. Identify two ways you can be a health resource person in your neighborhood.

7

The Team Concept of Community and Home Care

OBJECTIVES:

After completing this unit, you will be able to:

- Compare and contrast hospital and community health care teams.
- Identify comprehensive services provided in community and home care.
- Discuss goals of the community health care team.
- Identify the role of the nurse on the community health care team.

As a nurse or student, you have been a member of a nursing team, assigned to care for patients in a hospital or nursing home. The team probably included student nurses, RNs, LP/VNs, and nursing assistants. The larger health care team, in addition to the nursing team, included the physician, dietitian, laboratory technician, and perhaps the physical therapist, respiratory therapist, or others.

This unit will help expand your view of the nursing and health care teams; you will develop greater "peripheral" vision in the team concept of health care. The communities, as discussed in the preceding unit, require a greater variety of team members to assist them in managing health concerns. Guidelines to successful teamwork in community health and the nurse's place on the team will be discussed.

DEFINING THE COMMUNITY HEALTH CARE TEAM

The community health care team combines professionals from many disciplines plus technicians with a variety of skills, and volunteers, figure 7–1. In the hospital the health care team is designed around a specific health concern that has caused the patient to be hospitalized. Tests, medications, treatments, therapy, and nursing care are planned and implemented to remedy or improve the problem to the point where the patient can be discharged. Those health professionals and caregivers with the skills required to tackle this health concern become the patient's health care and nursing team.

The community health care team is expanded to assist the patient in completing activities for daily living at his highest level of functioning. This often requires comprehensive community and health care services. In addition to any necessary ongoing health care or monitoring, it means providing

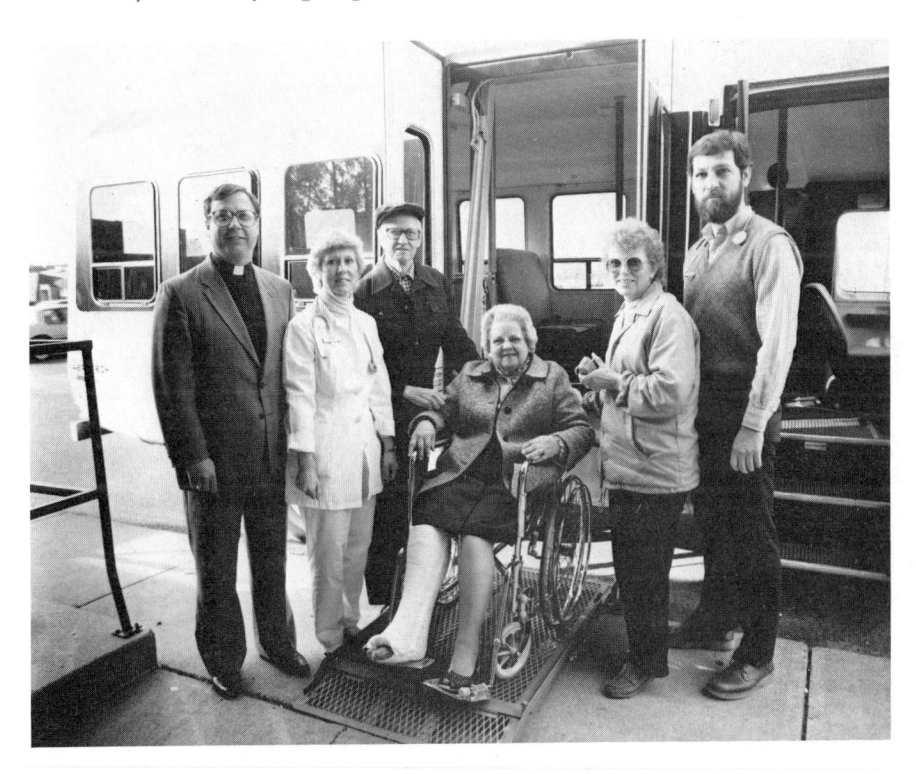

Figure 7–1 A community health care team

services to assist in areas indirectly affected by the health concern. This may include services to complete tasks in the home, transportation, interaction with the community as well as completion of personal care, figures 7-2 and 7-3.

Unit 8 will present a sampling of members of the community health team and the role and responsibilities of the members. To better understand this concept of care in the home and community, imagine the following situation.

Mr. Featherstone is a 72-year-old retired train engineer. He has been overweight most of his adult life and has a twenty-year history of essential

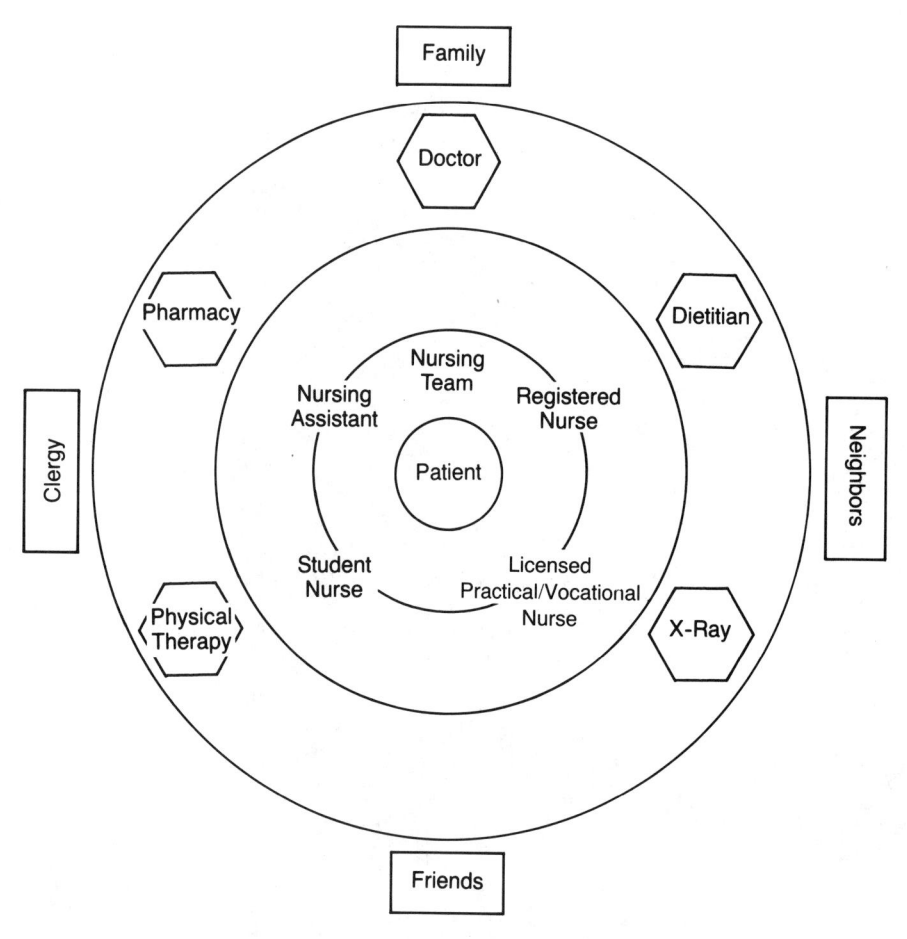

Figure 7-2 Hospital health care team

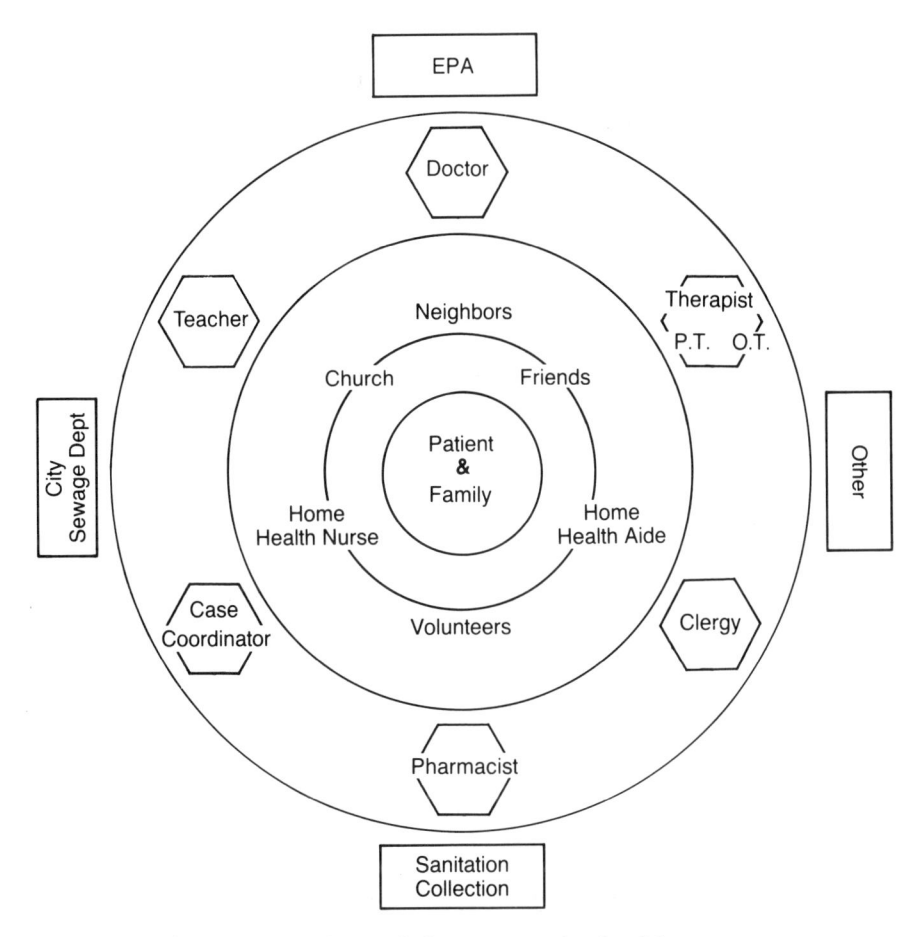

UNIT 7/THE TEAM CONCEPT OF COMMUNITY AND HOME CARE

Figure 7-3 Interactions of the community health care team

hypertension. One morning he awakes with tingling in his right arm and has difficulty buttoning his shirt. He ignores the problem, thinking that old age is gaining on him faster than he wants to admit. By lunch time he has difficulty with his soup and coffee; both tend to run out the corner of his mouth. His wife insists he see the family doctor.

Mr. Featherstone has had a stroke that affects his right side. In the hospital his condition is stabilized. The health care team in the hospital includes his family doctor, a consulting neurologist, the dietitian, laboratory, radiology, and pharmacy personnel. The nursing team is primarily concerned with assessing the effects of the stroke. They are taking his vital

> **KEY CONCEPT: DEFINITION OF THE COMMUNITY HEALTH CARE TEAM**
>
> - Includes professionals from many disciplines
> - Includes technicians and volunteers
> - Assists the patient in completing activities for daily living
> - Helps the patient achieve his highest level of function

signs and doing neurological checks frequently. The next matter for consideration is the prevention of complications. The focus of the health care and nursing team is to diagnose his health problem, to prevent additional injury, and to provide treatment and care to improve or stabilize his condition so that he may go home.

After one week Mr. Featherstone is dismissed on oral anticoagulant therapy and a 1200-calorie low salt diet. He has considerable weakness on his right side, but has gained some strength each day. His doctor suggests short term home health care to the Featherstones and an agency nurse visits them the day before dismissal from the hospital. Discharge planning has begun with the Featherstones, their family doctor, the hospital nurses, and the home health case coordinator.

In the hospital the case coordinator for Mr. Featherstone reviews discharge orders and plans for rehabilitation. The patient's environment, previous schedules, and activities are considered. Since Mrs. Featherstone doesn't drive, transportation is arranged to get Mr. Featherstone to his doctor appointments. A repair or maintenance service is contracted to install railings by the stairways. Their church organizes volunteers to take Mrs. Featherstone to the grocery store once a week. The agency contracts with a home care physical therapist to provide physical therapy three times a week and teach Mrs. Featherstone how to do passive range-of-motion exercises. The case coordinator assigns a home health nurse to reinforce the teaching of the hospital dietitian. With Mrs. Featherstone, the nurse reviews typical meals and discusses the sodium content of canned and boxed food on hand.

As recovery continues, the home health nurse assesses the progress of Mr. Featherstone's recovery and his wife's ability to assist. The nurse continues to monitor blood pressure, the effects of drug therapy, and the strength and use of the extremities. Plans are made for the day when the Featherstones will not need the nurse's guidance or the other services of the home health agency. The case will then be closed.

DEVELOPING A COMPREHENSIVE HEALTH CARE TEAM

There is no blueprint for developing a comprehensive health care team. As stated in the preceding unit, it is often difficult to associate persons or communities with health risks. There is no prescribed method to identify and evaluate a problem. The situation is similar in developing a team to assist people to manage health concerns.

Two basic approaches to coordinating comprehensive services will be considered here. The first one is viewed from the health risk. In situations such as natural disasters, the American Red Cross has plans to mobilize and provide food, clothing, and shelter. Government agencies have the responsibility to test drinking water and evaluate other health threats. Utility companies and community services have emergency plans ready. In other situations where a population at risk has been identified, less formal services are provided. Some examples are the monthly blood pressure screenings held in elderly apartment complexes, health fairs, and diabetic screening in shopping centers.

The second approach is to develop a comprehensive health care team from the position of the person at risk. This can be confusing and frustrating. There is no basic home care plan for stroke victims that Mr. Featherstone can refer to when he goes home from the hospital.

There is no single point of entry for receiving services from the community health care team. Mr. Featherstone entered through the hospital health team. Referrals often come from clergy, school teachers, neighbors, formalized support groups, and other concerned persons. Sometimes home care agencies, health departments, or other agencies are called directly by the patient or family. Other times physicians or clergy are called upon for help. Too often situations become desperate before help is obtained. The family may be trying to cope without help, or are unaware of the available services. (An example could be a family caring for a member with advancing Alzheimer's Disease.)

Whatever the approach in identifying the need for comprehensive health care services, there are criteria for deciding who should be on the team: (1) specific needs of an individual or group should be identified and priorities established; (2) the services required to meet the need are identified; (3) the persons needed to implement the plan are selected. The complexity of the problem and the degree of knowledge and skill required will help determine the type of service and staff that is needed.

> ### KEY CONCEPT: DEVELOPMENT OF A COMPRE-HENSIVE HEALTH CARE TEAM
>
> - Identify a health risk to the community or target population.
>   Identify and involve community members with the skills to tackle the health concern.
> - Identify a patient with a health risk.
>   Identify and involve community members with the skills to help the patient achieve his highest level of function.

IMPLEMENTING SUCCESSFUL TEAMWORK

Since your first clinical student experience, you have read, discussed, and been involved in the team concept of providing patient care. You may not have been aware of the specific ingredients, but you could "feel" when the process was really teamwork and when it was not.

Some of the ingredients that made teamwork successful during the clinical experience are similar in the community health care team: good communication, knowledge of the tasks and limitations of self and others, and mutual respect for patients and team members. The following will be helpful to you as a community health team member.

- Learn the characteristics and responsibilities of other services and caregivers. Agencies may have job descriptions or resource information, like hospital policy manuals. Libraries and government agencies are good resources for learning more about other professions and services.
- Continue to develop communication skills. Begin with having confidence in your own abilities and respect other team members for theirs. Sharpen your speaking, listening, and writing skills. Ask for feedback! Resources to improve these skills can be found in community continuing education classes.

- Focus on the group process. Individual members may work independently but are a part of the group. The group leader—as well as the rest of the team—must exhibit knowledge, skills, and a positive attitude. To continue in successful group work, members need motivation, ongoing feedback, and positive reinforcement. Abilities of the members need to be matched with the appropriate tasks.

    Successful groups have structure and standards. The structure identifies the leader or persons responsible for coordinating tasks to meet goals. It also identifies lines of communication between members. Standards are rules. They indicate acceptable levels of performance. Taking community education classes in group dynamics may be helpful if you are part of a comprehensive health team.

- Be committed to the team concept. Team effort requires a cohesive group. Working as a group affects the performance of individuals as well as the team. If you have been a member of a team that did not run smoothly, perhaps someone was not committed to the team concept. This person wanted to "do their own thing" or "go their own way."

KEY CONCEPT: IMPLEMENTING SUCCESSFUL TEAMWORK

- Learn characteristics and responsibilities of other services and caregivers.
- Develop communication skills: speaking, listening, writing.
- Focus on the group process.
- Be committed to the team concept.

REACHING THE GOAL OF THE COMPREHENSIVE HEALTH CARE TEAM

The goal for the comprehensive health care team is to assist or provide services to a person or group in order to achieve and maintain the highest level of function possible. This is a holistic approach that includes physical, emotional, and spiritual comfort and well-being. It is more than the absence of illness. Two methods are: (1) promoting individual wellness, and (2) promoting health education.

Promoting Individual Wellness

Each profession or service with similar tasks has specific objectives in their efforts to manage or remedy health concerns. The physical therapist employed in home care evaluates and assists patients who have a musculoskeletal disorder. The goal is to achieve the highest level of function possible, to complete the activities of daily living.

Emergency vehicles and services provide rapid transit and technical life support systems from the patient's home to an acute care center. Buses or vans for the handicapped or senior citizens provide door-to-door service for transporting people to work, an appointment, or another destination. These vans have motorized lifts for wheelchairs and other specialized equipment. The goal is to help this population group maintain their highest level of function in the community.

These are a few examples of community services that, when combined, provide for a comprehensive community health care team. Planning and implementing goals may be jeopardized by problems. A common one is poor communication. Problems can occur because of inadequate information, wrong channeling of information, and the absence of feedback.

Uneven distribution of services may be another problem. Unit 2 covered this issue in relation to the number of health care professionals available to the population in urban and rural areas. This lack may also occur within community services. Urban populations may have a variety of sources of public transportation, while rural citizens may have one or none. The variety in the metropolitan areas may lead to the problem of duplication of services. The city may have special buses equipped for handicapped riders, volunteer agencies may have grant monies to provide the same service, and private business may set up similar services for profit. Although there is duplication of services in some situations, there may be gaps in others. For example, in most cities Meals-on-Wheels service is provided to shut-ins from Monday through Friday. This means there are some people who do not have a meal on weekends.

There can also be problems associated with rules and regulations. As the nation and world become more sophisticated with technology, more paper work is required. Professional caregivers and agencies have specific regulations for licensure. The scope of practice that the license allows must be followed.

Promoting Health Education

Earlier units discussed how the cost of health care has been responsible for changes in the present health care delivery system. In the past most health care education and money were focused on curative measures. At this time the focus is moving toward health promotion and healthy lifestyles. The workplace is beginning to expect employees to be more responsible for their health. The government is considering legislation that rewards citizens when they take care of their health and expects them to pay a larger percentage of the bill when they do not. More choices will be made by the consumers. For example, the person with a small fracture of the distal tibia may have the choice of an air splint or a lower leg cast. The woman with a malignant breast cyst may have the choice of a lumpectomy and radiation, or a mastectomy and no radiation. These choices must be informed choices, figure 7–4.

Community health team members promote health education by being knowledgeable resource persons. Those at the grass roots level are alert to hazards to community health. They can clarify technical language, present information to community groups, and give consulting services to other community health team members.

The media is the primary source of the public's health education; this includes television, newspapers, and magazines. Information may be presented in special reports, documentary dramas, and public participation campaigns. Informal polling reveals that a low percent of the population

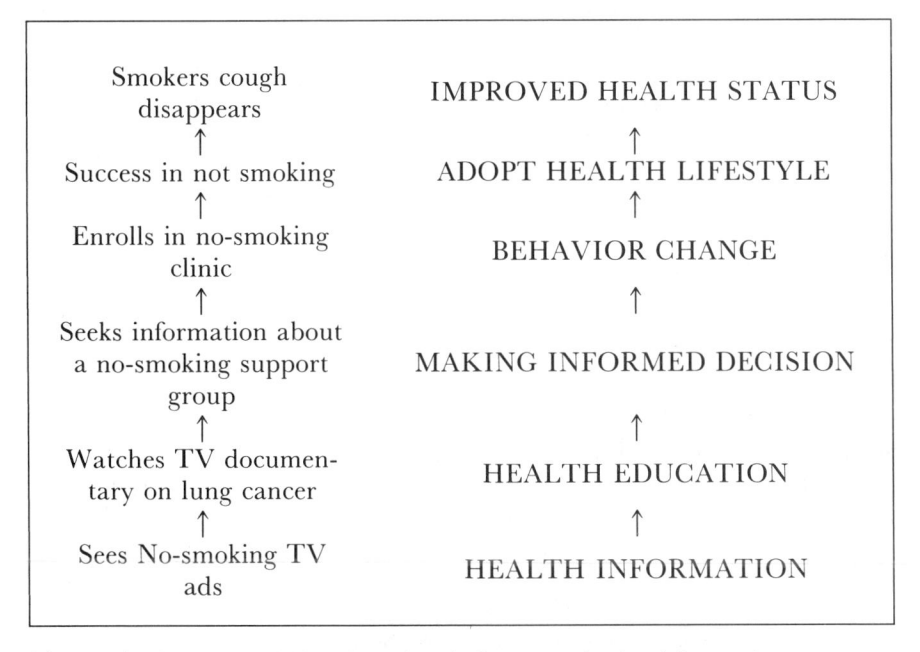

Smokers cough disappears ↑	IMPROVED HEALTH STATUS ↑
Success in not smoking ↑	ADOPT HEALTH LIFESTYLE ↑
Enrolls in no-smoking clinic ↑	BEHAVIOR CHANGE ↑
Seeks information about a no-smoking support group ↑	MAKING INFORMED DECISION ↑
Watches TV documentary on lung cancer ↑	HEALTH EDUCATION ↑
Sees No-smoking TV ads	HEALTH INFORMATION

Figure 7–4 How public education influences the health continuum

voluntarily uses automobile seat belts. Accidents (all types) are the major cause of death to children. In the summer of 1986 a television station and newspaper in Minnesota began Project Lifesaver. The goal was to remind the public of safety hazards when driving and to reduce fatalities during holiday weekends. There were 38 fewer fatalities in 1986 than in 1985.

KEY CONCEPT: METHODS TO HELP REACH THE HIGHEST LEVEL OF FUNCTION

- Promote Individual Wellness—Coordinate a network of services to allow anyone to achieve or maintain the highest level of function.
- Promote Health Education—Be a good resource person for health information; direct individuals to reliable sources that help them to make choices.

IDENTIFYING THE NURSE'S ROLE

As a member of the nursing team in the hospital you may have been primarily concerned with the physical problem that brought the patient to the hospital. You were alert to the need for using sterile technique in changing a surgical dressing. You assessed fluid intake, elimination, and independent ambulation as a part of the postoperative routine. The environmental hazard that concerned you most was nosocomial infections. You washed your hands over and over! You were not as concerned about other environmental factors, such as lighting and ventilation, since they are controlled by government and hospital regulations.

As a member of the comprehensive community health team, however, your assessments will be broader as you develop that "peripheral vision." Your hands-on care will consist of the same skills. You will be taking vital signs in the patient's home, in the doctor's office, in a storefront clinic, or during a preschool health screening. During these times of direct contact with people, you will utilize your senses of looking, listening, feeling, and smelling. You will also be alert to other health concerns expressed by the person such as, "I would come to have my blood pressure checked more often, but I don't have a way to get here." You will be a community resource person, connecting people and services to provide the highest level of functioning possible.

In the home you will be more alert to environmental safety. Is the home well ventilated? Is the lighting adequate? Are there any loose rugs or other items that may cause falls?

KEY CONCEPT: COMMUNITY ROLE OF THE NURSE

- Expand patient assessments to all areas of daily living.
- Practice usual nursing procedures in expanded settings.
- Become more alert to environmental safety.

SUMMARY

Health care services are provided in a variety of community settings. Health is viewed as the highest possible level of functioning and not just absence of illness. Health education is becoming a higher priority to assist the public in making choices about their health maintenance. Health promotion and care is more of a cooperative effort. We no longer take our bodies to the hospital to be fixed like we take our automobiles to the garage to be left for the mechanic. We are becoming more informed and responsible.

Doctors, nurses, dietitians, and others are using the same knowledge and skills that they have in the past, but they are implementing them in a variety of settings. They are working cooperatively with services that they have not worked with closely in the past. For smooth teamwork, caregivers need to be more aware of the characteristics and responsibilities of other services in comprehensive health care. Nurses continue to provide direct patient care as they expand their assessments to identify community sources to help their patient toward the highest functioning level possible.

FOR DISCUSSION

- Visit with a laboratory technician, physical therapist, or other health team member who has provided services in the home or community setting. Do they see their job as the same or different from their job in the hospital?

- Interview a paramedic, driver of a bus for the handicapped, sanitation worker, or other comprehensive health team member. How do they view themselves and their work in promoting health and preventing health risks?
- What comprehensive community health care services are available in the community where you live?
- Reflect on a patient you recently cared for in the hospital. What community services would be required for this patient to function at his highest level when at home?

QUESTIONS FOR REVIEW

1. Describe how the hospital health care team is organized to meet patient needs.
2. Describe how a community health care team could be designed to meet the needs of a patient who will receive care in his home.
3. Identify a characteristic of successful teamwork.
4. Discuss a goal of the community health care team. (Consider transportation, nutrition, or community interaction.)
5. How is the role of the nurse on the community health team different from the role on the hospital health team?

8

Community and Home Care Team Members

OBJECTIVES:

After completing this unit, you will be able to:

- Discuss role changes of the nurse in community and home care nursing.
- Identify the role of three non-nursing health team members in community and home care nursing.
- Discuss the relationship of family assessment to community and home care nursing.
- List three cultural factors that could influence implementing community and home care nursing.

This unit will help you to compare and contrast the role and responsibilities of the nurse in the traditional institutional settings and in community and home care, figure 8–1. The role of doctors, therapists, family, and other team members in the expanded settings will be discussed and examples presented.

Home care or outpatient care is not appropriate for every situation. The health care delivery system, as you learned in Section One, is exploring and evaluating the best setting for specific health concerns and population groups. Nurses and other health team members will adapt their skills to assist in all these areas.

To practice in these expanded settings means that you will be working within a broader, more varied comprehensive health care team. This was discussed in the previous unit. It also means that you will be implementing

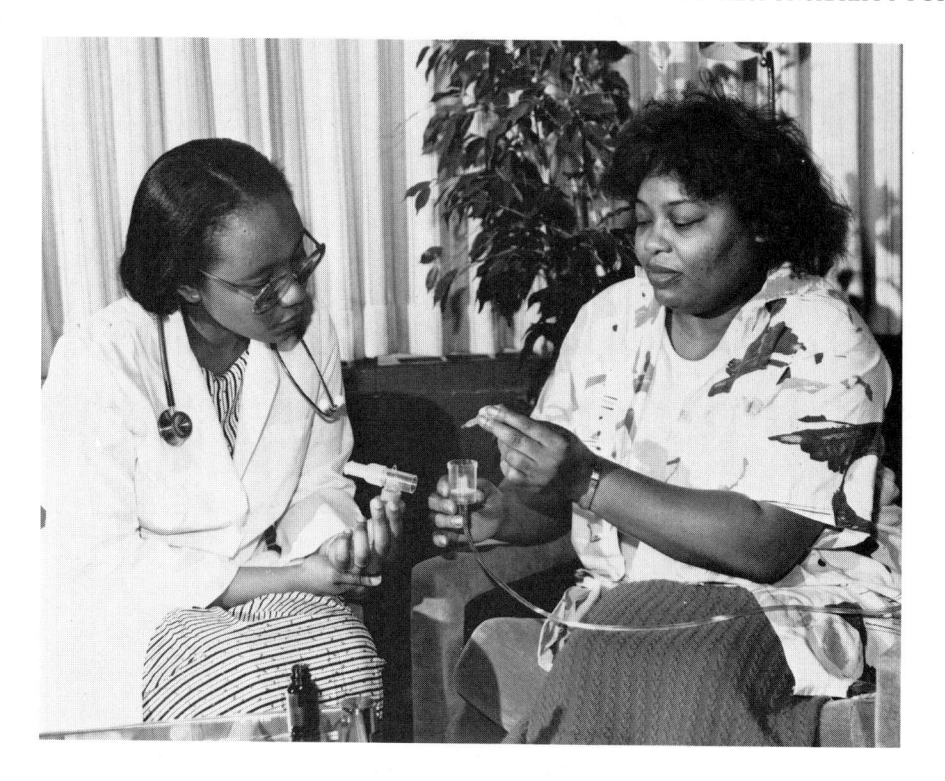

Figure 8–1 Home health patient learns to use a nebulizer.

your tasks more independently. You will be required to be more autonomous and make independent decisions. Today, nurses who have practiced in a hospital for many years may become employed in a home health agency. Many of these nurses comment that independent decision making was their biggest adjustment. Nurses have made and do make independent decisions and are good problem solvers. But traditionally there have been other nurses and team members across the hall, or back at the nurses' station, to "compare notes." Reference books and other resources are at their fingertips. Traditionally, nurses have consulted with others during all steps of the nursing process. This has been primarily for reinforcement and continuity of care.

The understanding of cultures and traditions is more integrated into nursing care in the community and home. When admitted to the hospital, the patient unconsciously compares it to a voyage to an unknown planet! Hopefully the stay is of short duration, almost everything familiar has been left behind, the surroundings are strange, and he doesn't understand the language. It's not his Turf!

Patients who receive home health care comment that the feature they like best about this approach is that they remain in control of the situation. They can usually plan their care, with the nurse case coordinator, around family routines and personal preferences. They can eat familiar food, maintain all or part of their family role, and continue with habits and customs. They can even sleep in their own lumpy bed!

During the study and discussion of this unit you should reflect on your own values and traditions. They will influence your approach and attitudes in assisting patients. Mutual respect is a key to successful patient rapport.

You have begun to focus on community health concerns outside of the hospital and the health team members that address and manage those concerns. In this unit you will focus on a variety of team members.

The doctor directs the health team in the hospital. The patient is admitted to the hospital with a medical problem that requires the doctor's orders for treatment. The type of treatment indicates the skills required and the appropriate team members; these members are followers of the medical treatment leader.

In the home care setting, the patient is the leader. There are times when a family member or another person may assume the leader role. The doctor, nurses, and other health team members then function as guides in managing total patient needs. The focus is on the patient rather than on the medical problem.

A patient receiving home care may have a stabilized medical problem while requiring continuous long term home care. He or she requires periodic check-ups with the family doctor just like you do.

IDENTIFYING TEAM MEMBERS AND ROLES IN HOME HEALTH CARE

A sampling of the comprehensive community health team members and their roles will assist you in comparing and contrasting the roles in the hospital and community.

The Patient

The patient is the most important team member and needs to participate as a team member for the group to meet their goals. It may be necessary to inform the patient about participation and individual as well as group responsibilities.

To make informed decisions about care, the patient may need additional information. Sometimes it's a brief lesson in anatomy and physiology such as how heart changes could make the feet swell. Another example is providing information about paying for rented equipment. This may assist the patient in understanding the reimbursement system.

Some patients may refuse to participate as a team member. Until now they may have been involved only in a passive role. Perhaps they deny they are ill or need help, their religious beliefs interfere, or their fears and pride prevent them from asking questions. A language barrier or medical jargon may get in the way. They may have a general distrust of the medical system.

The patient DOES have the right to refuse care and assistance. Health professionals legally and ethically must have the patient's cooperation and consent to proceed with community and home care.

The Family

The family becomes the second most important member of the team since they are usually the primary caregivers. They also need to realize they are a part of the team and must be committed to the team effort. Tasks specific to the caregiver role must be learned. For example, they may be taught how to position a paralyzed patient in bed, using pillows and other supportive devices. These health team members must go the extra mile as this role is added to the tasks of homemaker, breadwinner, or parent.

Family members may hesitate or refuse to be a part of the team for some of the same reasons the patient refuses. They may live too far away to be an active part of the team and are able to provide only emotional support by letter or telephone. Differing views and attitudes may make them unwilling to participate as team members.

Traditionally the definition of family has referred to parents and their offspring. Today's society broadens the definition to include persons sharing a caring bond. This may be a group of people sharing the same apartment or household. An extended family may include children living with an aunt and uncle. A nontraditional family can include caring neighbors and friends who share in family tasks and concerns.

The Doctor

Since the patient is more often the leader in the community and home care team, the doctor assumes the role of one of the patient's guides in health maintenance. The doctor may be a co-leader with a patient recently dismissed from the hospital. Examples would include those patients requiring more medical management with medications, laboratory studies, or wound care.

Most doctors involved in home care are family practitioners. Specialists are usually consulted when the patient has an acute problem. Their time with patients is often intermittent or of short duration. Patient progress is then monitored by the family doctor.

Commitment to the community and home care concept is required by doctors, too. They need to move from the illness care concept to the health maintenance concept and view other comprehensive health team members as peers.

Some doctors have resumed making "house calls." This practice almost disappeared in the 1950s. Some believe the tradition should never have stopped. It was in the home that the doctor could assess the patient's environment. Often the real root of the problem could be determined. Today many family doctors say that over half of the patients they see in their offices are there for psychosocial reasons. The patient makes an appointment to have a blood pressure reading and get a prescription renewed because of his need to talk to the doctor.

The Nurse

In community and home health care, the nurse practices in all levels of health intervention: health promotion, primary prevention, curative intervention, and maintenance and rehabilitation. The greatest growth area of nursing practice in each level is in patient and family teaching. Figure 8–2 shows a home health nurse teaching a patient's wife how to monitor her husband's pedal pulse with a Doppler instrument.

Providing instructions and explanations to the patient has always been the first step in bedside care and all nursing procedures. But the nurse has been a part of 24-hour care and continual monitoring. The community and home health nurse must turn that control over to the patient. That may not be easy for nurses who learned and have practiced the illness model; it emphasized nurse control over patient care. Now the focus is on the nurse as a teacher, guide, and cheerleader.

In addition to the expanded settings you are learning about, nurses are being employed in diet and nutrition clinics, health clubs, and other settings. Here nurses may provide formal or informal health teaching. Factories and offices are employing more nurses for the health services, wellness, and fitness programs.

The nurse in the community health team must be a generalist. In the doctor's office and in home health care, patients you will meet will be of all ages with health concerns affecting any body system.

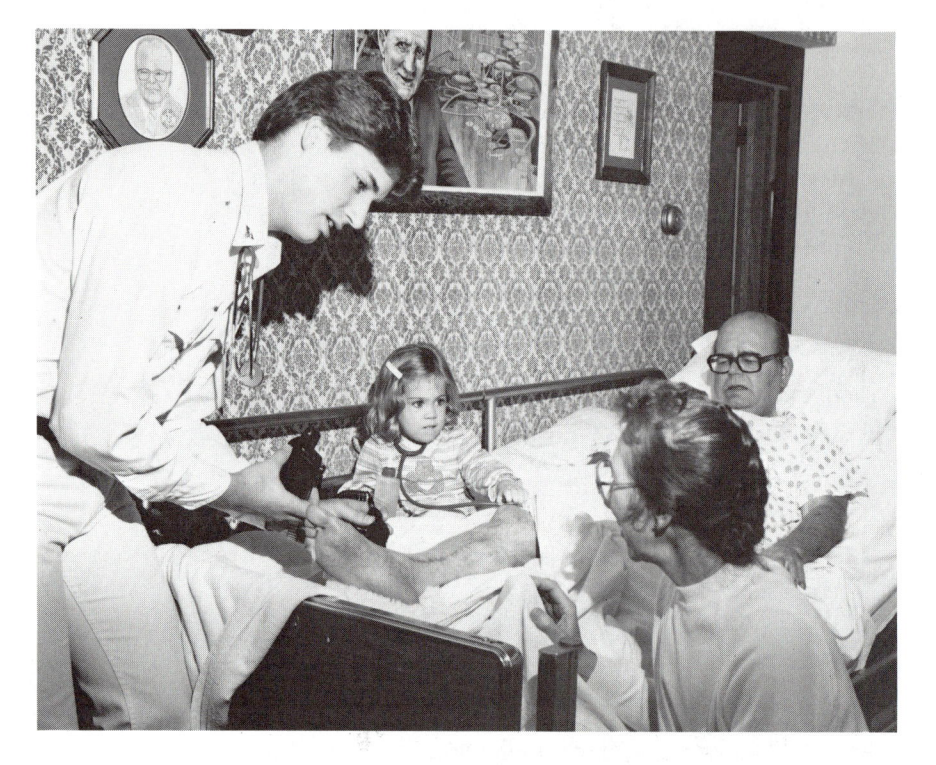

Figure 8–2 Home health nurse teaches a family member.

The Homemaker and Home Health Aide

This community health care worker is employed by home care agencies and works exclusively in the patient's home. A person may be employed as a homemaker or home health aide or the position may include the combined tasks.

The homemaker completes light housekeeping tasks such as vacuuming, sweeping, dusting, laundry, and meal preparation for the patient and family. The home health aide provides personal care such as bathing and dressing and assists with activities of daily living. The role and responsibilities are similar to the nursing assistant in the hospital or nursing home.

These health team members are frequently recruited from the neighborhoods in which they are to be employed. They are acquainted with the customs of the neighborhood. This promotes comfort in the patient and the home health aide. The homemaker and home health aide provide a link between the patient and the case coordinator. Because of their unique place in the neighborhood and on the health team, they may be able to contribute information that other team members cannot.

Life experiences of homemaking, caring for family members, and being involved in the community are often the educational background for these team members. Some have a wealth of knowledge and insight. Many home health aides adapt their patient care skills from previous hospital or nursing home employment. In some states a formalized class has been implemented to teach homemaker-home health aide skills. In Minnesota the Department of Health has developed a 60-hour class. This class is offered primarily in vocational schools. Many home health agencies employ persons who have completed this course.

The Neighbors, Friends, and Community Volunteers

These community health team members have greatly expanded roles and are involved primarily with persons receiving home care. When a person is in the hospital, neighbors and friends are visitors. Sometimes they may provide a meal for family members, water the plants, or bring the mail to the hospital.

In home care the expanded roles may include providing some of the direct care in place of the family member, providing transportation to doctor's appointments, or assisting with homemaking tasks.

Community volunteers are frequently organized through churches, support groups, and senior citizen centers. They are sometimes, but not always, more involved in home care when family members are not present or available to assist. An example is a handicapped child who may require many hours of exercise and stimulation every day. Often friends and neighbors learn these skills to provide respite for the parents. Area Agencies on Aging, through the Older Americans Act, have the Retired Seniors Volunteer Program (RSVP). Senior citizens volunteering with this group provide a variety of services, including being foster grandparents and companions to the homebound.

The Clergy

Ministers, pastors, priests, and rabbis have always been involved with their communities. In home health care they may be providing more personalized and direct spiritual and emotional care to the patient and family. They may also be a liaison between the patient and other health team members. The patient may view the clergy as less threatening than doctors, nurses, and those assisting with physical care. The elderly may be more willing to discuss emotional problems with a minister they know than with a psychiatrist they don't know.

The Teacher

Teachers are in the position of observer not too unlike the bedside nurse. The teacher interacts with students on a continuing and intermittent basis. This provides the opportunity to identify health status and concerns as well as to promote good health practices.

In home health care the teacher is often a tutor for the homebound student. These may be children with trauma such as extensive burns or multiple fractures that may require long term home care. With tutoring, the student will be able to continue with peers upon returning to the classroom. Some large school districts have teachers contracted specifically for tutoring. It is an advantage to the patient and family if the student's regular teacher is able to be the tutor. The teacher is then a liaison between the patient and class members at school. This communication provides emotional support for the patient and family. As a community health team member this provides the continuity needed in comprehensive health care.

The Dietitian

Dietitians provide consultation about diets and nutrition in numerous settings. In recent years nutrition has become a greater focus in all levels of health intervention. The dietitian may be a guest speaker for a support group, nurses in continuing education, or an industry wellness group. Case coordinators in home care will consult with a dietitian when a patient is having difficulty tolerating or accepting a diet. Perhaps this might be a follow-up procedure in hospital discharge planning. The patient's doctor could order a home visit by a dietitian.

Dietitians are also employed to plan menus for meal programs. An example is the congregate dining program for senior citizens. Some dietitians are developing independent practices.

The Pharmacist

The pharmacist's role as a resource person has expanded considerably in recent years. Drug research and therapy has become more complex. More information is available on medication side effects and interaction with food and beverages. Patients are becoming more knowledgeable about the action and the side effects of medication they are taking.

As a member of the community health team, the pharmacist instructs patients on their medications when a prescription is filled. They answer questions when the patient calls the pharmacy. As home care expands, more pharmacies may provide a service to deliver prescriptions to the home.

The Social Worker

Social work, like nursing, is concerned with the person's highest level of functioning. As a community health team member, the social worker practices in many settings. At times the role of the social worker and nurse overlap. One example is the role and responsibility of the case coordinator. Depending on the focus and philosophy of the home care agency, case coordinators may be nurses or social workers.

Another role as a community health team member is that of working with groups who have social problems. Some of the target populations for which social workers implement therapy programs are: abusers and victims of abuse of alcohol and drugs; abusers and victims of physical abuse of children, elderly, and spouses; those who are suicidal; and mentally handicapped. The victims, as well as family and friends, are involved in group sessions.

Social workers may be coordinators of day care or respite programs where personal interaction is a key objective.

The Therapist

Occupational, physical, and speech therapists have also expanded their responsibilities from the hospital to the community health care team. Some are employed by hospitals that have expanded their services to home health care. These team members may have patients who are hospitalized and may visit others in the home. Extended care and rehabilitation facilities also employ these therapists.

With the current change that promotes early hospital discharges, a patient may not be ready for therapy until he has gone home. Some therapists have established independent practices and then are contracted by home care agencies. Some agencies employ the therapists as part of their staff.

Like the nurse, the therapist incorporates more patient and family teaching in their practice. A physical therapist may teach a mother and other family members certain exercises to assist the child with cerebral palsy. Suggestions for adapting the home to meet the child's needs can be given.

A speech therapist will teach an aphasic patient's wife how to support her husband's efforts to relearn speech. In the role of resource person, the physical therapist may be a guest speaker at an arthritis support group and the speech therapist can be invited to speak to a stroke or laryngectomy support group. See Table 8-1 for a review of health team members' role changes in community health.

Table 8-1 Health team members role changes in community health

TEAM MEMBERS	EXPANDING ROLE
Patient	has more control of own care, increased responsibility for own health and illness care
Family	may be primary caregiver
Doctor	guides patient in health maintenance
Nurse	practices at all levels of health intervention increases patient teaching transfers control of care to patient
Home health aide	adapts personal care skills from traditional care settings
Friends, Neighbors	actively participate in supporting family care; provide respite to family
Clergy	is liaison between family and health team
Teacher	tutors home-bound patients
Dietitian	is consultant in independent practice, discharge planning for patient diets
Pharmacist	resource for medication information increases home delivery service of prescriptions
Social Worker	serves as coordinator of day care, respite care group work for families with problems
Therapists	teaches patient and family to participate in care establishes independent practices

An Example of Home Care

The example of Rico Sanchez will examine the needs of a person requiring long term care from the community health team.

Rico is a 35-year-old bookkeeper who works with a fast-food chain. He had been drafted the summer after he graduated from high school and sent to Viet Nam. He suffered multiple wounds, including a spinal injury. After months of hospitalization and rehabilitation in a Veterans Hospital, he returned home to his parents, brothers, and sisters. He was confined to a wheelchair. With government funding he enrolled in the community college and, upon graduation, decided he was going to make it on his own.

Through veteran groups, Rico was established with a case coordinator. He was able to rent an apartment designed for disabled living. A special van transports him to and from work every day. A homemaker home health aide comes two hours twice a day to assist him with personal hygiene and light housekeeping. Some of his co-workers come on their days off and all go by van to the grocery store and shopping center. Buddies from his days in the VA Hospital come frequently for an evening of music and conversation. Rico's home health nurse comes every two weeks to evaluate his overall status. His urinary catheter is checked and changed if necessary. The results of daily passive range of motion exercises is evaluated. The key to Rico's health maintenance is the prevention of potential complications.

KEY CONCEPT: ROLE CHANGES IN HOME HEALTH CARE

- Patient and family become more directly involved in decision making and caregiving.
- Doctors, nurses, and other health team members become guides and teachers of care.
- Friends and neighbors are more active in assisting the patient and family.

CULTURAL INFLUENCES ON HEALTH CARE

In the introduction of this unit you learned that the hospital environment is a unique community with a culture of its own. When entering this environment, the patient leaves many traditional practices, either consciously or unconsciously. The desire to be a "good patient" and do things "their way" is stronger.

When the patient remains at home to receive care, traditions and practices are maintained. The nurse and other health team members must, in most situations, assist the patient with health concerns within the boundaries of cultural and social traditions. The nurse's experiences, traditions, and attitudes will also affect the view of the patient, environment, and needs. Accepting persons for who they are is vital in community health nursing.

Reviewing objectives and goals will help the nurse to keep on target with the responsibilities in home care. A patient's home may appear cluttered and disorganized to you, but if your directions to complete the foot soak and apply a sterile bandage were followed, the objectives are being met. However, if the nurse identifies obvious health risks, then health teaching must be done or the situation be reported to the case coordinator for appropriate intervention. When spoiled food is found in the refrigerator, the food should be discarded. If uncollected trash is attracting rodents, the case coordinator or agency should be notified so appropriate community services are contacted.

The following examples of special concern will guide you in expanding your assessment skills. They will encourage you to focus on your own views and values. Finally, they will assist you to place the patient's needs and focus of care within his framework.

The Patient's Beliefs About Health

How a person defines health and health care has a great influence on the pursuit of health care and compliance with the suggested intervention. One person may consider himself well if he "feels okay" and is able to complete his daily tasks. He may feel that the absence of illness is wellness. Another person may believe that health care means frequent check-up appointments to the dentist, eye doctor, foot doctor, and other specialists. These visits to doctor's offices may seem as commonplace to them as routine grocery shopping.

Some people believe in home remedies or fad treatments advertised in a magazine. There are two predominant influences on a view of health: one is the attitudes and practices of parents or those responsible for health during childhood years; the other is experience. People will return for health care if they feel good about a previous experience. The health care facility met their needs. The nurses, doctors, and other health team members answered their questions and made them feel comfortable. If an experience was not pleasant, they are reluctant to return unless it's absolutely necessary.

Nontraditional Health Practices

Nontraditional health practices are usually considered to be those that operate outside traditional medical practice of the time. They may not follow currently accepted scientific principles. But times change and so does the acceptance of nontraditional therapies. Until recent years acupuncture was not accepted as a method of treatment in the United States. Now it is practiced in hospitals and clinics for pain management. Biofeedback and hypnosis are also becoming accepted by the public and medical community.

Some nontraditional health treatment methods are utilized successfully along with accepted medical treatment. Others may be practiced by quacks. *Quacks* are persons who claim to have cures but have no foundation for their apparent knowledge and skills. Often their incentive is financial gain. People who feel desperate for miracle cures from cancer or other conditions are often the targets of quacks.

Nurses practicing in clinics and home care will be confronted with nontraditional health practices. The initial reaction may be negative because of the strong traditional medical framework of nursing education. The nurse needs to use good problem-solving techniques to determine if the patient is being harmed. Are these practices interfering with the traditional medical practice also chosen by the patient? A clinic or agency team conference may be the best place to discuss the situation. Perhaps the patient needs more information. The bottom line is that the choice belongs to the patient, not the nurse.

Some samples of nontraditional health practices are: acupuncture, biofeedback, chiropractic, faith healing, homeopathy, and hypnosis. A brief discussion of each method is presented.

Acupuncture. The Chinese have practiced acupuncture for 5000 years. It is based on the belief that man echoes nature. The human anatomy and physiology is aligned with the seasons, elements, climate, and time of day. The seasons and months of the year are either Yin or Yang and their delicate balance is homeostasis. When homeostasis is not present, the acupuncture needles are used to restore the balance. The decision of where to place the needles is based on the complex theories of the practice.

Currently the major use of acupuncture and acupressure in the United States is in pain management such as in lumbar disc syndrome. In acupressure the thumb and forefinger apply pressure to designated parts of the body.

Biofeedback. This practice employs techniques whereby a person obtains feedback or messages from different parts of his body. It is believed that health can be controlled entirely through the power of the mind. In the training process the person learns how to read personal body signals and then be able to control involuntary functions such as temperature and blood pressure.

Currently biofeedback has been successful in treating patients with migraine headaches and premenstrual syndrome (PMS). In clinics where more diagnostic procedures are being done, patients are instructed in the relaxation techniques of biofeedback. Procedures such as an endometrial biopsy can be completed without medication.

Chiropractic. Chiropractic therapies may no longer be considered nontraditional, but they are not practiced in traditional settings of the hospital or medical clinics. All fifty states now license chiropractors, but they cannot perform surgery or prescribe drugs. The name, chiropractic, comes from a Greek word meaning "done by hand." Manipulation of the spine is based on the principle that vertebral dislocation is the cause of many problems.

Home health nurses may visit patients who are seeing both chiropractic and medical doctors for the same complaint. However, the patient may not wish to share that information with either doctor!

Faith Healing. Belief in a higher being, in the self, and in the power of the mind is recognized by all health practices—including traditional medicine. You may have seen how the will to live has affected the progress or outcome of an illness.

Generally a person who practices faith healing believes that the power to heal has been received from God. He believes the remission or cure is caused by the healer.

Christian Science believes that disease is more a matter of the mind; unhealthy thoughts cause disease. Treatment involves devotion, study, prayer, and the practice of believing that the ailments are illusions.

Homeopathy. Homeopathy is based on the "law of similars." The belief is like cures like. If a substance produces specific symptoms in a healthy person then it will be the remedy to cure an ill person with the same symptoms. Homeopathic remedies are developed from animal, vegetable, and mineral sources. They are usually given in dilute amounts with only a trace of the original substance and are called "energized medicine." Homeopathic doctors are usually medical doctors who have become interested in this method of therapy.

Hypnosis. The practice of hypnosis has been in existance for centuries. Through the power of suggestion hypnosis may affect a person's behavior or reaction to physical stress. It involves a state of consciousness rather than a state of physiology. How it works is not clearly understood, but that it does work contributes to the understanding that there is a psychosomatic nature to health.

People seek hypnosis therapy for behavior-related problems such as weight control and smoking. Hypnosis is used by some doctors for their patients during labor and delivery.

Socioeconomic Status

The socioeconomic status of the patient or family has a great impact on their seeking health care and in continuing with recommended therapies.

There are many ingredients in the socioeconomic picture. They may include money, family background, education, field of work, and accomplishments at work and in the family group. The neighborhood in which one lives places him or her in a social setting of expected behaviors. There may be an unwritten "dress code," speech pattern, and other behaviors. Whether a woman obtains prenatal care from a family practitioner or an obstetrician may be a part of the expected social behavior in the neighborhood.

The greatest socioeconomic influence in a patient's health care is employment. Being employed and having health care benefits most often influences whether or not a person or family will seek medical attention. The exception is a life-threatening situation.

The economic crisis of midwestern farmers in the late 1980s forced many to make drastic family budget cuts. Some chose to drop their medical insurance policies. They would have to ignore health problems or turn to government assistance.

Other Cultural Influences

Language, ethnic background, religion, and nutritional practices are some other cultural influences that the community and home health nurse may encounter. They will be a part of the care plan.

The use of non-English language needs to be considered. Often in bilingual families English is spoken at school or work, but the native language is spoken at home. It is an advantage for the nurse working in a clinic, home care, or other community setting serving clusters of ethnic groups to know local languages.

Clinics and other community agencies need to consider employing nurses, technicians, or volunteers from the neighborhood. They will understand all aspects of the lives of the patients from the area. The need for bilingual health education materials should be identified.

Nurses working in schools with classes for deaf students will benefit by being able to do signing. *Signing* is a method of communicating ideas with specific hand and finger movements. Signing classes are frequently offered in community adult education classes. Health education materials in Braille should become more available for the blind.

Being aware of how a language is used is equally important. Within the English language the use of words within different generations and in many geographic settings varies more than most of us realize. Always ask for clarification and feedback of messages.

Another language, of course, is "computerese." The need for nurses to understand computer printouts and to key in information is expanding. You will need to explain coding and other basic information to your patient. You may be the first to see his bill when you arrive on his doorstep as his home health nurse.

Everyone is a member of a culture or ethnic group. There are beliefs, values, practices, and biases within every group. Often we do not realize that many of these traits are "preprogrammed." They are adopted by subtle behavior and suggestion from our parents, grandparents, and others in everyday living.

Religion is tied very closely to a person's ethnic group and health beliefs. Some knowledge of the religions of the neighborhood where the nurse is practicing will help in understanding the role that it plays in the patient's health. The nurse may learn about these religious practices by reading or attending services. If asked, patients often are quite willing to share basic beliefs of their faith.

Food habits are probably the most firmly established characteristic of a culture. They are very difficult to change. They have been shaped and practiced for generations. You may have observed this in an elderly patient who is suppose to adjust to a new diabetic diet.

Food plays a major role in social activities and religious festivities. In many cultures specific foods are associated with specific illnesses, with pregnancy, and rites of passage through age groups.

The nurse needs to be keenly aware of this cultural influence. The goal is to balance cultural preferences with therapeutic diets and good nutrition.

Health Care of Ethnic Peoples of Color

There are dozens of distinct ethnic population groups in the United States. Since the term "ethnic" does not refer to skin color, "people of color" is used to describe people who come from groups with a skin color other than white. In the United States, the largest groups of ethnic peoples of color are the native Americans, Asians, black Americans, and Hispanics.

Second or third generations of immigrants may know and practice little of their heritage or may be closely tied with traditions. Stereotyping should be avoided by nurses since the practices of individuals in a family may vary more than those of differing ethnic groups.

Native Americans The native Americans (American Indians) comprise less than one half of one percent of the U.S. population. Health care risks with this group are related primarily to environmental and economic status. Many native Americans live in overcrowded housing and are economically disadvantaged. They may have limited access to health care. Specific health concerns include otitis media in young children and upper respiratory conditions, such as influenza and tuberculosis, in adults. The Indian Health Service was organized in 1955 to focus on preventive health measures and provide comprehensive health care.

Nurses and other caregivers need to be aware that this group values privacy. The family is very important and may be broadly defined to include an entire community of native Americans. Some groups are matriarchal and others patriarchal, which may influence the consent for care. Communication with caregivers is generally not a problem.

Asian Americans This population group includes Chinese, Japanese, Filipinos, and Southeast Asians. Many came to the United States for industrial jobs and with the dream of all immigrants to have a better life. For many the dream did not come true due to low pay. This condition results in substandard housing and inadequate nutrition. The Chinese came in the 1800s to help build railroads. The Filipinos were recruited to work on farms and plantations. More recently Laotians, Cambodians, and South Vietnamese emigrated to escape political oppression.

The Asian Americans have often received inadequate health care. Specific health concerns are hypertension, tuberculosis, and bone disorders. Some of the people prefer their traditional medicine and do not seek modern health care.

Caregivers should realize that this population group strongly values social manners of privacy, respect, and courtesy. The family unit is very important, and caring for the ill is considered a family and community responsibility. Language barriers must be considered in planning nursing care. Within the Asian American population there may be many languages with many dialects.

Black Americans In the United States the black Americans are the largest group of ethnic people of color. This group comprises almost 12 percent of the population. Black Americans continue to struggle to overcome discriminatory practices that have historically followed them. The first blacks in the United States did not come by choice, but as slaves.

Health concerns include those related to poverty and nutrition. There is a high infant death rate, hypertension, diabetes, obesity, heart disease, and malnutrition.

Caregivers should realize that historically, black families have been affected by poverty and discrimination. Establishing trust is vital in caregiving since the act of trust has been violated so often. Communication should not be a problem if the usual clarification and feedback techniques are implemented.

Hispanic Americans Hispanic Americans include Spanish-speaking people from Mexico, Puerto Rico, Cuba, Central and South America, and Spain. This group is now about five percent of the United States population. Many live in the Southwest. The Spanish settled this part of the United States. Some Hispanics came as political refugees and others as migrant workers.

Health concerns are those related to economic disadvantages. These include obesity, diabetes, hypertension, and respiratory conditions. Nutritional deficiencies are related to low economic status.

Nurses need to be alert to communication problems in planning care for patients of the Hispanic culture. There are many dialects and the patient may fear an English-speaking caregiver. Hispanic patients look to their family for support. Family honor is valued and families tend to be patriarchal. Communication is expressive and touch is welcomed.

KEY CONCEPT: CULTURAL INFLUENCES IN HEALTH CARE

- How the person defines health and health care
- Nontraditional health practices
- Socioeconomic status of patient or family
- Beliefs, values, and practices of ethnic groups
- Use of non-English language
- Food habits

FAMILY INFLUENCES ON HEALTH CARE

We are all products of our environment: the air we breathe, the city where we live, and the kind of work we do. Our family, or the people we have lived with as children and as adults, has a great impact on our values and traditions.

The home health nurse, as a member of the community health team, is a grass roots observer of the family unit. This nurse is in the home for a period of time on an intermittent basis and is able to see how the environment and interactions of the family members affect the wellness or illness of the patient.

The clinic nurse is also an observer in a less direct role. Members of a family have periodic office visits and telephone inquiries are made. A nurse who is a keen interviewer, listener, and observer is able to collect much data. Nurses who are involved in day care, respite care, and other extended health care delivery settings will interact more closely with the patient and family.

The following overview of the family system will assist you in assessing the family interactions and the patient's environment. Problems of abuse will be reviewed. The nurse should recall that there are many variables in the network of family systems. These include ethnic origin, religious influences, social class, part of the country where they live, and other variables. You are encouraged to seek continuing education classes to learn more about the beliefs and traditions of the families you will assist in your nursing practice.

Family Structure

In most cultures the family is considered the basic social unit. Each person assumes roles as an individual and as a part of the group. The structure of the family is the interrelationship of all the roles of each family member. These roles have expected and accepted behavior patterns. In addition to mother, father, daughter, son, and breadwinner, there can be favorite daughter, clumsy son, athlete, family clown, lazy good-for-nothing, workaholic, and countless other roles. Each person can have many roles with expected behaviors. They may have asked for the role or have been given it. They may or may not realize they have the role; it can be healthy or harmful.

Families have perimeters and gates. The family *perimeter* is a boundary or limit to which they will extend membership. In some families the perimeter encircles only the parents and children. Others draw in a variety of people with "open arms" and continue to extend beyond the boundaries. The gate may be restricted to only approved marriages or as liberal as all known relatives or any friend in need. Open families accept all members, new members (by birth, adoption, marriage), and their ideas. Closed families are exclusive to their own members and ideas. Many families fall in between open or closed. Those on the extreme ends may have problems. The totally open family may be vulnerable to unhealthy outside views and actions. Existing problems may be aggravated in the closed family. The members' roles may be cloudy or overlap and change at times. At times of illness responsibilities may be shifted from one member to another.

The family exists and grows as members depend on and interact with each other. This fosters the socialization and culturization of the family.

Families have typical norms that often follow traditions of previous generations or are a result of experiences such as education or travel. Examples of norms are eating habits, social behaviors, and expected achievements in school (report cards, or participation in sports). These norms provide guidelines for members' feelings and attitudes. Sometimes whole cultures are shaken with shifts in roles and norms.

An example of cultural change is the women's movement. Some adults have grown up in a family where there was much sharing of tasks and overlapping of roles. They may not be concerned with roles being identified as male or female. For example boys and girls in the same family, who shared the tasks of mowing lawns and washing dishes, may feel comfortable sharing these tasks in later years with a husband or wife. However, adults who grew up in families with well-defined tasks for men and women may feel uncomfortable interchanging these tasks.

Another part of the family structure includes verbal and nonverbal communication patterns: who talks to whom about what. Does each member interact freely with other members? How are children included? Are children "seen and not heard"? Are there communication conflicts? For example, is someone discussed as if he or she is not there? Does one member communicate with another only through a third member? Often there are unwritten rules regarding accepted topics to discuss, such as sexual behaviors.

Families with an Acute Problem

When a crisis occurs, such as the diagnosis of advanced breast cancer in a young mother, the coping abilities of a family may be observed. Those with flexibility in their roles may adapt well. Families with more rigid roles may have continual problems with coping. The strength of the family structure, values, and socialization affect the coping mechanism. The social network and support system help individuals and families to survive a crisis.

Families with Problems

All families have problems. We hear about the generation gap and mid-life crisis. Children argue and siblings test their ideas, strengths, and their parents' patience! The process readies them for interactions and socializing in adulthood. Most families absorb "the good days and the bad days" into everyday life. When problems have grown to the point where the family is not functioning, then help is needed. The nurse must be aware of signs of a nonfunctioning family and report them to the case coordinator, a supervisor, or the doctor.

There are clues in observing families with serious potential problems. They include open or underlying tension. This may be seen as a breakdown in communication and a weakening in the trust and support system. Another clue is involvement in an illegal or counterproductive activity such as shoplifting, or dropping out of school. A third clue is a physical or economic problem that adversely affects all members of the family. This may occur when there is a job loss by the major wage earner or when family members cannot cope with an acute illness.

The nurse should also assess for social isolation. Is the family withdrawing from community involvement and neighborhood interactions? The last clue is for any sign of abuse or neglect to any member of the family.

In home health nursing, the nurse is not a therapist to families with problems. When the nurse has reported a clue to the case coordinator, additional data will be collected and the team will develop a plan. In addition to ongoing observations, the nurse's role in implementing the plan may be reinforcing patient education, being a positive role model, or being a good listener. Figure 8–3 presents clues to families with problems.

Abuse in the Family

There are many forms of physical and emotional abuse and neglect. In pediatrics class, you probably learned about child abuse. The vulnerable adult was studied in adult or gerontological nursing, and substance abuse in pharmacology or mental health classes. It is recommended that you review that information and be aware of specific laws and regulations in your state. Nursing continuing education classes are offered periodically to keep nurses current with new information.

Child Abuse. Child abuse has been prevalent for centuries, but laws against it are surprisingly recent. Now every state has a Child Abuse Law. The law defines what constitutes abuse or neglect, the age of those protected (usually those under 18), and who is obligated to report suspected cases.

Remember that child abuse may be seen in any social class or culture. It does tend to have a generational pattern. A child abuser was probably also abused as a child.

- Open tension: arguing, fighting
- Underlying tension: abnormal quiet, little interaction
- Breakdown in communication
- Weakening in trust and support system
- Involvement in illegal or counterproductive activity
- Physical or economic problem leading to family dysfunction
- Isolation: family withdraws from neighborhood, community
- Any sign of abuse or neglect

Figure 8–3 Clues to identify families with problems

An accident is not child abuse. Child abuse is not an accident. A caregiver should suspect abuse when there is evidence of an injury and the data conflicts with the information given by the parents or other person responsible for the child. See figure 8–4 for guidelines to physical assessment of child abuse.

Neglect may be detected by observing behavior. Also compare normal growth and development patterns of children with the child suspected to be neglected.

Parents or other caregivers should be observed for any subtle indication that they may be abusive. Clues may be obtained from comments about their childhood. What are their feelings about that time? What are their feelings about their parents' roles? Other clues come from the interactions with their own child. What are they expecting? Do they show affection? Do they discipline with a firm but gentle touch?

Nurses must be aware. Nurses must be the child's advocate.

Vulnerable Adults. Abuse and neglect of the dependent elderly is becoming more visible with the return of home health care. For years hospital nurses have suspected neglect with some elderly patients admitted to the hospital. Some of these patients have had fractured hips or acute congestive heart

SOFT TISSUE INJURIES
  BURNS–NEW OR OLD
  BITE MARKS
  BRUISES AND ABRASIONS
  LACERATIONS

  LOOP-TYPE LESIONS
    ON THE ABDOMEN OR BACK

GENERAL SIGNS
  POOR SKIN CARE
  SIGNS OF NEGLECT
  REPEATED INGESTION OF
    TOXIC SUBSTANCES
  MALNUTRITION

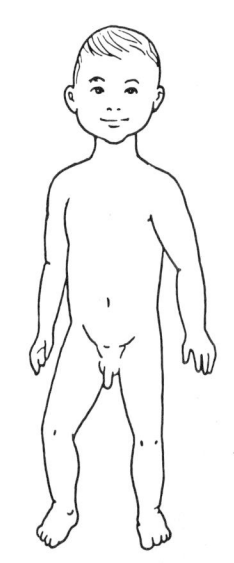

INJURIES TO THE HEAD REGION
  SECTIONS OF HAIR MISSING
  SCALP INJURIES
  SKULL FRACTURES
  RETINAL HEMORRHAGE
  INJURY TO DENTAL RIDGE;
    MISSING OR DAMAGED TEETH

PERINEAL AND GENITAL INJURIES
  BURNS IN PERINEAL AREA
  ABNORMAL DISCHARGE
  LACERATIONS

BONE AND JOINT INJURIES
  HEMATOMAS AROUND
    JOINTS
  PERIOSTEAL SWELLING
  EVIDENCE OF FRACTURES
    OF THE RIBS OR
    EXTREMITIES

Figure 8–4 Signs of child abuse (Reprinted, by permission, from Patricia A. Lesner, *Pediatric Nursing*, Fig. 17–1. Copyright 1983 by Delmar Publishers Inc.)

failure. Large deep decubiti or accumulated debris on the skin have been clues that the patient has not been assisted with personal care.

You have learned that in home health care the family is most frequently the primary caregiver. Adequate instructions, demonstrations, and other information will be given to the patient and family. If the patient care or progress is unsatisfactory, the nurse should consider the possibility of neglect. Sometimes the caregiver may be a substance abuser.

As you recall from earlier discussions, the United States was built on Federalism, or control by local government. In developing policy for the vulnerable adult, each state has its own legislation. See figure 8–5 for reporting abuse of the elderly in your state. Many states report suspected cases to the Department of Health, or Welfare, or other human service agencies. That will be the responsibility of your agency. As the nurse caregiver, you should report suspected abuse or neglect to the patient's case coordinator or your supervisor.

Substance Abuse. Substance abuse can include alcohol, illegal drugs, and prescription drugs. A single drug or a combination of drugs can be the cause. Abuse occurs when there is physical damage or when a pattern of dysfunction appears in activities of daily living. This dysfunction affects not only the person who abuses substances, but those around him or her. These include family members, co-workers, classmates, friends, neighbors and many others.

The nurse must be careful not to stereotype those who abuse substances. The alcoholic is not always the skid row vagrant. The heroin or cocaine user is not always a teenage runaway.

The alcoholic is generally well educated and a professional or is employed in a managerial position. Perhaps this was one of the incentives to consider alcoholism a disease and promote active rehabilitation programs. Many businesses today do not fire an identified alcoholic; they have recovery programs within their wellness programs.

Those abusing narcotics and other substances include doctors, nurses, professional athletes, entertainers, and many others. Public and private treatment centers are available. Most are located near larger metropolitan areas.

There is a nationwide effort to eliminate illegal drugs and to increase education about their negative effects. The increased use by young people is alarming. To some extent this is a product of our culture. Technology brings more and more to us in the time frame of "right now." We want gratification immediately and success tomorrow. Our emotional framework can't handle that and we look for crutches. However, the substances have been available for centuries and eliminating them may be an unrealistic goal. Improving access to educational information may be a more realistic

THE LEGAL SIDE

REPORTING ELDER ABUSE: A SUMMARY FROM THE STATES

STATE	Coverage FOR WHOM	PHYSICAL MISTREATMENT	MENTAL ANGUISH	NEGLECT	EXPLOITATION	OTHER ABUSES COVERED	Reporting WHEN	PENALTY FOR FAILURE	Investigation WHEN
Alabama (1)	18+ (impaired)	✔	✔	✔	✔		Immediate verbal, then written.	● ✹ ☼	Required within 3 days of report
Alaska (2)	65+	✔	✔	✔	financial		Within 24 hr.	●	To begin promptly; including personal interview *
Arizona (3)	(impaired)	✔		✔	✔		Immediate verbal, written in 48 hr.	●	As soon as possible.
Arkansas (4)	18+ (impaired)	✔	✔	✔	✔		Immediate verbal, written in 48 hr.	● ⊘	Not defined.
California (5)	65+	✔	✔	✔	✔	abandonment	Immediate verbal, written in 36 hr.	● ✹	Not defined.*
Colorado (6)	65+	✔		✔	✔	confinement intimidation	Immediate written.	—	Immediately if adult consents in writing.
Connecticut (7)	60+	✔	✔	✔	✔	abandonment	Within 5 days.	● ✹	Prompt evaluation, including home visit by ombudsman.*
Delaware (8)	18+ (impaired)				✔		—	—	Prompt and thorough.
Florida (9)	(impaired)	✔	✔	✔	✔		Immediate verbal, written in 48 hr.	●	Immediate.*
Georgia (10)	18+ (impaired)	✔	✔	✔	✔		—	●	Prompt and thorough, including a home visit.*
Hawaii (11)	65+	actual or threatened	✔	✔			Immediate verbal, then written.	—	Action toward preventing further abuse within 24 hr., when appropriate.*
Idaho (12)	60+	✔	✔	✔	✔	abandonment	Within 24 hr.		Prompt and thorough evaluation of report.*
Illinois (13)	60+	✔			financial		—	—	—
Iowa (15)	18+ (impaired)	✔		✔	✔		—	—	Adult to be examined in 1 hr. for immediate physical threat; otherwise, within 24 hr.
Kentucky (16)	18+ (impaired)	✔	✔	✔	✔		Immediate verbal or written.	● ✹	As soon as possible.*
Louisiana (18)	18+	✔	✔	✔	✔	extortion	Immediate verbal, then written.	● ✹ ☼	Prompt, including interview and home visit, if possible.

FOOTNOTES:

Reporting is voluntary, not mandatory, in four states: Colorado, Iowa, Wisconsin, Wyoming. Nine states have no "in home" adult-abuse reporting law: Indiana (14), Kansas (16), Maryland (20), Mississippi (24), New Jersey (30), New York (32), North Dakota (34), Pennsylvania (38), South Dakota (41).

▒ Physically or mentally impaired.
— Not specified.

• Consent required for services to allegedly abused elder.
☼ Report filed with department named in reference.
● Misdemeanor
✹ Fine, ranging from $25 to $1000
☼ Imprisonment, ranging from 10 days to 6 mo.
⊘ Civil liability for damages due to failure to report

Figure 8–5 Reporting elder abuse (Reprinted, by permission, from *American Journal of Nursing*, April, Vol. 85, No. 4. Copyright 1985 by American Journal of Nursing Company. "Reporting Elder Abuse: It's the Law" by Marshelle Thobaben and Linda Anderson)

STATE	Coverage	FOR WHOM	PHYSICAL MISTREATMENT	MENTAL ANGUISH	NEGLECT	EXPLOITATION	OTHER ABUSES COVERED	Reporting WHEN	PENALTY FOR FAILURE	Investigation WHEN
Maine (19)	18+	✔	✔	✔	✔		confinement	Immediate verbal, written in 48 hr. ☀	licensing board notified.	—
Massachusetts (21)	60+	✔						Immediately.	● ☀	—
Michigan (22)	18+	✔	✔	✔	✔			Immediate verbal.	◐	Within 24 hr.
Minnesota (23)	18+	✔	✔	✔				Immediate verbal, then written.	● ◐	Immediate.
Missouri (25)	60+	risk						—	—	Prompt and thorough.
Montana (26)	60+	✔	✔	✔	✔			—	●	—
Nebraska (27)		✔		✔				Verbal, then written.	●	Immediate if warranted by report.
Nevada (28)	60+	✔		✔	✔			Immediate verbal.	●	Within 3 days.
New Hampshire (29)	18+	✔	✔	✔	✔		confinement	Immediate verbal, then written.	●	Within 3 days.*
New Mexico (31)	55+	✔		✔	✔			Promptly.	●	Immediate.
N. Carolina (33)	18+	✔	✔	✔	✔			—	—	Prompt and thorough, including home visit.*
Ohio (35)	60+	✔	✔	✔	✔			Immediate verbal or written.	—	Within 24 hr. in an emergency, otherwise within 3 working days.*
Oklahoma (36)	65+	✔		✔		financial		Prompt oral.	●	Prompt and thorough.*
Oregon (37)	65+	✔		✔		abandonment		Immediate verbal.	● ☀	Prompt.
Rhode Island (39)	60+	✔		✔	✔	abandonment		Immediately.	● ☀	Immediate.
South Carolina (40)	18+	✔		✔	✔		confinement	Immediate verbal.	● ☀ ☼	Within 3 days.
Tennessee (42)	18+	✔	✔	✔	✔	✔		Immediately.	● ☀ ☼	As soon as possible. Reporter notified of determination.*
Texas (43)	65+	✔	✔	✔	✔			—	—	Within 24 hr.*
Utah (44)	18+	✔		✔	✔		confinement	Immediately.	● —	—*
Vermont (45)	60+	✔		✔	✔			Verbal, then written in 1 wk.	● ☀	Within 72 hr
Virginia (46)	18+	✔	✔	✔	✔		abandonment	Immediately.	—	Prompt, including home visit and consultation with relevant others.
Washington (47)	60+	✔	✔	✔	✔		abandonment	Immediate verbal, then written.	—	—*
West Virginia (48)	18+	✔		✔				Immediately.	● ☀ ☼	—
Wisconsin (49)	60+	✔		✔		material		—	—	Within 24 hr.
Wyoming (50)		✔		✔	✔			—	—	—

Figure 8–5 (Continued)

route. This view supports the health continuum of providing health information that directs a person towards choices for improved health.

The health focus continues to move towards wellness. Increased information about side effects of medications is available. There is a tendency to avoid medicating unless necessary. There still continues to be misuse and abuse of prescription drugs. The home health nurse needs to be aware of the patient's medications, actions, and side effects. Untoward symptoms in the elderly may be the result of repeated doses due to forgetfulness. They do not recall taking the medication and take it again.

See figure 8-6 for clues of substance abuse. If you suspect substance abuse, report it as you would other abuses. It is easy to make excuses for the patient or family member. If you have established a rapport and trust relationship, reporting abuse may not be an easy task.

With all suspected forms of abuse, follow agency and state guidelines carefully. It is the nurse's responsibility to report objective signs of abuse. Generally the abuse or neglect takes place on private property. Be aware of personal liability.

- preoccupation
- change in personality/behavior
- hiding/protecting supply
- loss of efficiency
- incomplete perceptions
- isolation
- rationalizing
- projecting
- blaming
- violation of values
- same time of day for use
- loss of control

Figure 8-6 Clues to identify substance abuse

> ### KEY CONCEPT: FAMILY INFLUENCES ON HEALTH CARE
>
> - Family Structure—how a family works and communicates as a system or network
> - Acute or short term problem in family—coping abilities and support systems assist through crisis
> - Families with problems—long term problems leading to a dysfunctioning family unit
> - Child Abuse
> - Vulnerable Adult
> - Substance Abuse

SUMMARY

Today more health care is being provided in the home and in community settings. Nurses are following this trend and practice in these expanded settings. To do this you need to become aware of changing roles of health team members.

In home health care you are a guest in the patient's home. The patient has more control in the schedule of the plan of care. Family, friends, and neighbors become involved in activities that help the patient to achieve and maintain his highest level of functioning in the community. Traditional health team members become teachers and guides in care.

You will need to understand cultural and ethnic influences on your patient's care. Beliefs in health care, including nontraditional health practices, will influence attitudes and participation in traditional medicine. The patient's financial and social status will influence whether he seeks health care. It will also determine where and from whom he seeks the care.

How a family operates as a group, with the roles each member has, determines the strength of its structure. In times of stress the coping abilities of members and the group may test the strength of the family system. When families are dysfunctional with problems such as abuse, they need outside help.

As a nurse in community and home health care you will continually collect and report data. You will collect data about services provided in the community to share with your patients and other members of the comprehensive health care team. You will collect data about your patient and his environment to report to your case coordinator or supervisor. Then the appropriate services and health team members can be involved with the patient care.

FOR DISCUSSION

- Interview someone in your class, school, or community who has a cultural background different from your own. How do your values about family, holidays, work or leisure time differ?

- What nontraditional health practices are available in hospitals or clinics in your community or neighborhood?

- Visit a clinic providing health care for ethnic peoples in your community. Are there doctors, nurses, or other health team members of that background employed there? Do they speak the native language?

- Do you know the laws in your state for identifying and reporting child and elder abuse?

- Visit a treatment center for substance abuse in your community or neighborhood. What specific services are available?

QUESTIONS FOR REVIEW

1. Identify two nonnursing health team members. Compare and contrast their roles in traditional and home health settings.

2. Define two nontraditional health practices that a nurse may encounter in home health nursing.

3. Discuss two cultural influences that need to be considered in a home health care plan.

4. List three characteristics of family structure that may influence coping mechanisms during a health crisis.

SECTION THREE

NURSES AND THEIR PATIENTS IN THE COMMUNITY

Unit 9   Adapting Basic Nursing Concepts to Expanded Settings

Unit 10   Applying Basic Concepts to Practice in Expanded Settings

Unit 11   Nurse's Responsibilities to Self and Career

Unit 12   Nurses' Influencing Future Health Care

Section Three transports the nurse who has developed an understanding of the health care delivery system and the community health team concept into practice in expanded settings.

Nurses will be guided to adapt known nursing concepts and skills to the expanded settings. Assisting patients with personal care and implementing treatments to improve health status is not new to nursing practice. Practicing this nursing care in the patient's bedroom or living room and beyond is new to the nurse generalist.

The section continues with a review of the nurse's legal and ethical responsibilities as a caregiver and as an employee. In the final unit nurses are challenged to influence future health care.

9

Adapting Basic Nursing Concepts to Expanded Settings

OBJECTIVES:

After completing this unit, you will be able to:

- Explain how use of the Nursing Process changes outside of the traditional setting.
- Discuss the importance of examining all of the patient's basic needs for data collection.
- Identify three key health concerns of two age groups.
- Discuss the importance of communication skills.
- Recall how the patient's family and culture affects health care.
- Discuss the importance of patient education.

Many concepts are taught in nursing education. This unit will review some of them and discuss how they are adapted when you practice outside traditional settings. You may need to refer to your basic nursing textbooks to review some of these ideas.

USING THE NURSING PROCESS

You will recall that the Nursing Process involves four major parts: assessment, planning, implementation, and evaluation. It is a continuous process, figure 9–1.

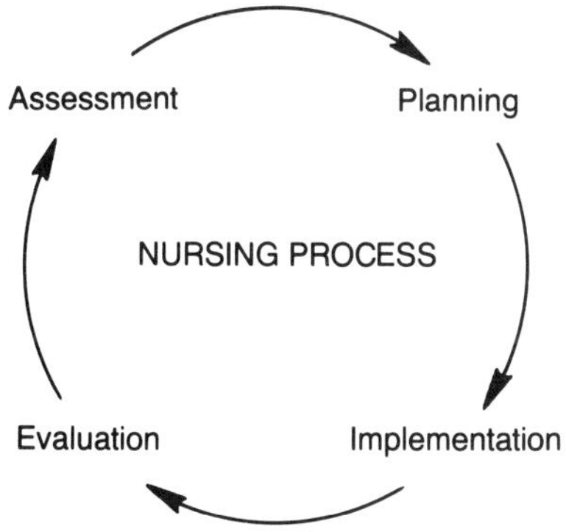

Figure 9-1 Continuous cycle of the nursing process

Assessment

Assessment is the first part of the Nursing Process. It must begin with data collection, or making observations, figure 9-2. This is one of your most important responsibilities. You have learned many ways to gather information. In the hospital you make observations, measure vital signs, read charts of all types, and talk with other caregivers.

In other situations, you may need to expand your horizons and stretch your observation skills. In home health care, you need to observe the living environment, family interactions, relationship of neighbors, clergy and other support persons—as well as make the usual observations about the patient. Much of this data is necessary to help plan the care you will be giving. Other caregivers will also need the data for their part of the care. The physical therapist may come weekly, but you may observe the patient's progress with exercises on a daily basis. You cannot focus on one problem only, but must view the patient as a whole person, part of a family and community.

If a patient comes to the clinic with an open sore on a toe, for example, you will have to think farther than whether or not his shoes fit properly. Perhaps he is a diabetic, perhaps he dropped a hammer on his toe, or perhaps he does not wash his feet very often. The initial interview should yield as much information as possible, so that the nurse practitioner or physician can treat him appropriately. Your thoroughness will save time for others.

The second part of assessment is the *analysis* of the collected data. The data is just a collection of facts; the analysis is the meaning you give those facts. This is also called "rationale." If the patient with the sore toe is unemployed, unkempt and thin, you may need to think about more than

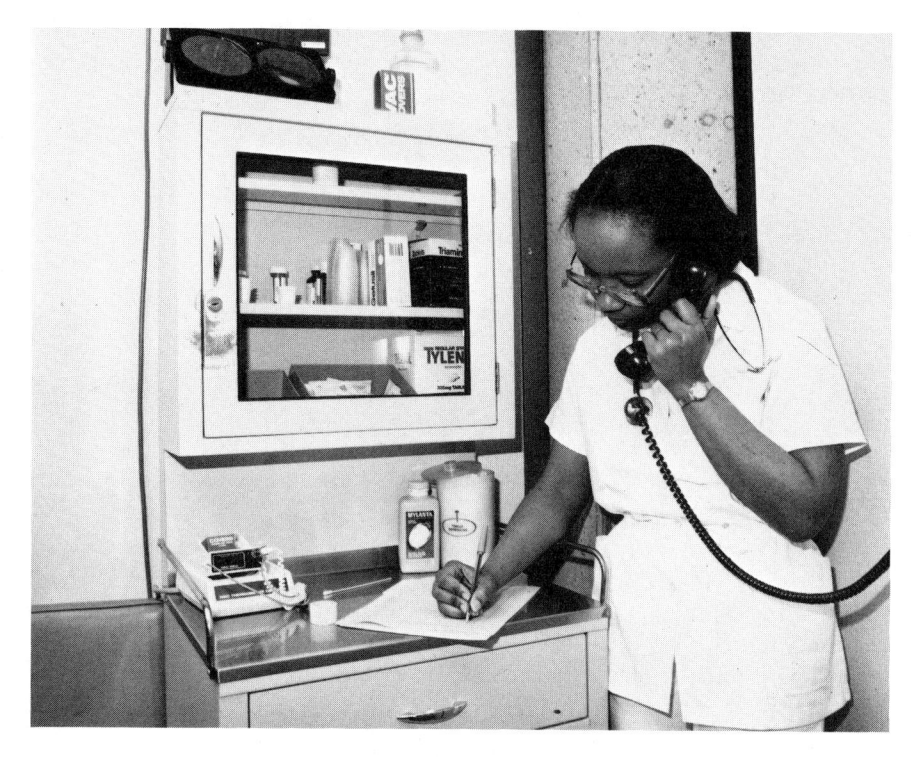

Figure 9–2 A nurse uses the telephone to collect patient data.

his toe. Perhaps he needs some review of basic hygiene. Remember that the presenting complaint may not be the only problem.

The purpose of the assessment section is to arrive at a *nursing diagnosis*, which is the problem to be addressed by the nurse. Data collection and rationale will lead you to a nursing diagnosis. Nursing diagnoses accepted by the North American Nursing Diagnosis Association (NANDA) are listed in Appendix A. Using a diagnosis from the list and individualizing it to your patient makes planning care more easily understood by all caregivers.

Planning

The second part of the Nursing Process is *planning*. In the hospital setting, you have participated in planning patient care. Nursing care conferences are held with various members of the nursing team (RNs, LP/VNs, student nurses, nursing assistants) to help make the care plan. Sometimes the report given at the change of shift may be used as a planning time.

In other settings, you may have other health workers to help you plan care. This could include the physician, physical therapist, social worker or mental health nurse. In a clinic, the physician or nurse practitioner may be responsible for planning care. You may then be delegated a part of the care.

You also need to include the patient and the family in planning. In hospital settings, procedures and treatments are often scheduled according to routine or for the nurses' convenience. In home health care, however, treatments should be scheduled according to the family's preference whenever possible. Perhaps your visit for changing a colostomy bag should be scheduled before the young children return from school.

Teaching the patient and family more about self-care is often part of the plan. You will often be assigned to do or review a portion of this teaching.

Implementation

Implementation means carrying out the plan of care. This is the "doing" portion of Nursing Process. Adapting the actual care to a different setting is not difficult. In the hospital you have a well-supplied linen room and access to special equipment. Each room has equipment for the patient's personal care; giving a bedbath is part of your routine.

Is giving a bedbath in the patient's home so different? The bed may not be adjustable, and the linen may not be folded just so, but the patient still needs a bath. A large bowl or a dishpan can be used as a basin. If the patient will require bedrest for a lengthy time, a hospital bed can be rented or loaned. The bath time can be used to explain, make observations, and give care just like you always have done.

If it is necessary to review self-care with the patient, the implementation will include that aspect of teaching. One way to begin is to ask patients to tell you what they already know about their illness. Then you can be sure they understand and you can add whatever information is needed. Maybe the patient can explain how he uses the glucometer for testing his blood sugar. Your interest and questions will help clarify the process. It will also help you identify when he is ready to continue learning.

Evaluation

The fourth part of the Nursing Process is *evaluation*. Evaluation is often done with the group that was involved in the planning. This always requires collecting more data to see whether or not the plan was effective. Again, this is where your observation skills become vital. Whenever possible, the patient should be included in evaluating progress.

Evaluation may have different outcomes. You may discover that the problem was solved, or you may find that a new problem has occurred. Consider again the patient with the sore toe. You explained the importance of regular foot care, but after ten days the toe is not healing. The plan was not effective and a new plan will be needed. Maybe the patient has trouble seeing his feet clearly. The new plan may include another family member to assist with foot care.

It is important to remember that the Nursing Process never ends, because the data you collect for evaluation becomes data for reassessment, figure 9–1. Table 9–1 compares the use of the Nursing Process in traditional and expanded settings.

Table 9–1 Nursing process compared and contrasted between traditional and expanded settings

TRADITIONAL SETTING	EXPANDED SETTING
ASSESSMENT	

Data Collection
  Objective Data:
    • chart, kardex, reports
    • frequent observations
    • reports from other nurses and specialty areas
	• may or may not have prior chart or care plan
	• often lengthy time span between observations

Subjective Data:
    • client complaints
    • family concerns
	• nurse interviews patient more thoroughly to obtain data

Rationale: • based primarily on objective data	• based more on subjective data • nurse needs interview skills
PLANNING	

Influences:
  • doctor's orders
  • institutional schedule
  • nurse's time
  • rules and regulations
  • unlimited supplies
	• doctor's orders
	• patient preference
	• priority needs
	• available supplies

Rationale: • more regimented, routine	• more flexible • nurse needs creative skills

Table 9–1 Nursing process compared and contrasted between traditional and expanded settings (Continued)

TRADITIONAL SETTING	EXPANDED SETTING
IMPLEMENTATION	
Focus:	
• nurse initiated	• nurse or patient may initiate
• minimal patient participation	• intent is maximum patient participation
• use standard equipment	• improvise with home supplies
Rationale:	
• nurse completes task	• nurse encourages patient toward independence
EVALUATION	
Focus:	
• nurse initiated	• nurse and/or patient may initiate
• short-term process; hours/shift/day	• may be short or long-term process; day/week/month
• ongoing	• ongoing
Rationale:	
• often based on nurse's goals	• based on patient's goals

CONSIDERING THE PATIENT'S BASIC NEEDS

Abraham Maslow's *Theory of Basic Needs* is used in many nursing programs as one approach to total patient care. Figure 9–3 illustrates one way that Maslow's theory has been adapted to nursing. You will see that physiological needs such as oxygen, food, and shelter must be fulfilled before the person can move on to higher needs of self-esteem. This is true whether or not the patient is in the hospital.

The hospitalized patient with asthma, for example, does not care about local politics if she cannot breathe adequately. Her first concern is getting enough oxygen. When her condition stabilizes she may show some interest in current events.

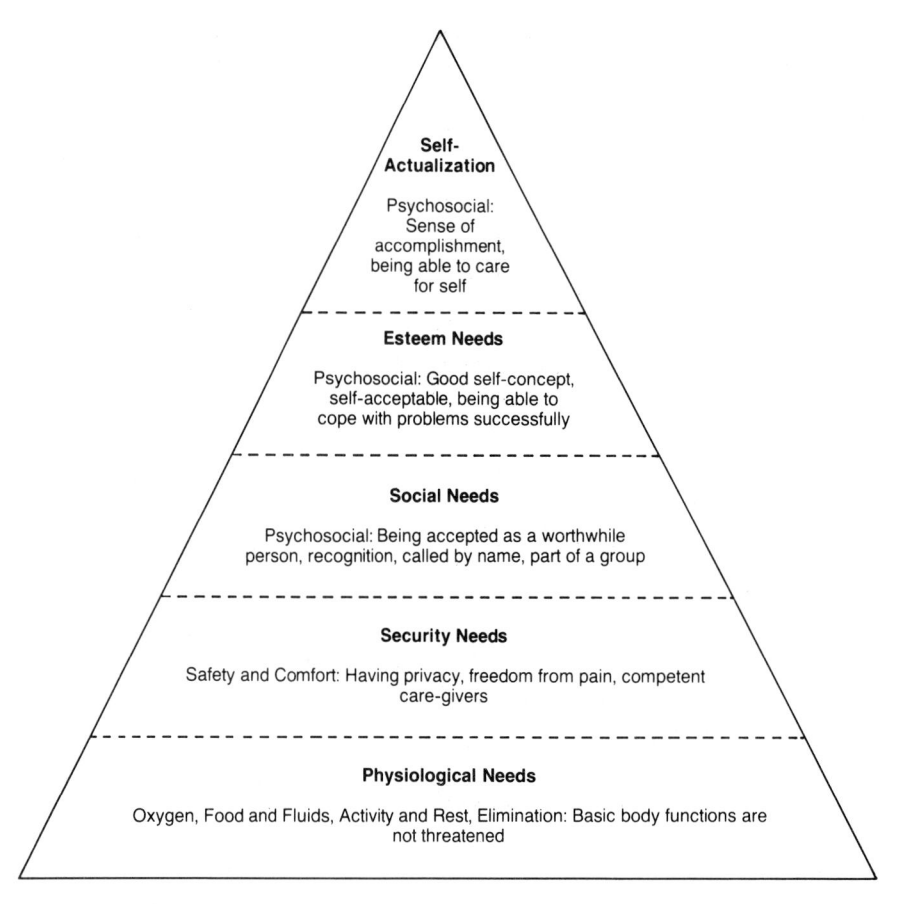

```
                    /\
                   /  \
                  / Self- \
                 /Actualization\
                /Psychosocial:  \
               / Sense of        \
              / accomplishment,   \
             / being able to care  \
            /     for self          \
           /------------------------\
          /      Esteem Needs        \
         /Psychosocial: Good self-concept,\
        / self-acceptable, being able to   \
       /   cope with problems successfully  \
      /--------------------------------------\
     /            Social Needs                \
    /Psychosocial: Being accepted as a worthwhile\
   / person, recognition, called by name, part of a group\
  /------------------------------------------------------\
 /                  Security Needs                        \
/Safety and Comfort: Having privacy, freedom from pain, competent\
/                        care-givers                              \
/------------------------------------------------------------------\
/                      Physiological Needs                          \
/Oxygen, Food and Fluids, Activity and Rest, Elimination: Basic body functions are\
/                              not threatened                                      \
/_____\
```

Figure 9–3 Maslow's hierarchy of needs adapted to nursing care

The young, single mother you meet at a well-baby clinic may appear very caring with her infant. But if she doesn't have enough food to eat, she won't be ready to hear about the baby's need for social stimulation. Table 9–2 uses a sample to show how needs are met a little differently in home health care than in a hospital.

IDENTIFYING CHANGES THROUGH THE LIFE SPAN

Erik Erikson's theory of developmental changes that occur throughout the life span is another concept that many nurses have learned. You may wish to review the ages and stages in another reference.

Table 9-2 Adapting care to meet basic needs

NEED/CONCERN	TRADITIONAL SETTING	PATIENT'S HOME
OXYGEN		
1. Supplemental oxygen ordered	Administer via wall, or tank	Agency contracts with supplier Nurse teaches procedure
2. Environment, temperature, ventilation	Institutional control	Family control Nurse assesses for special need, checks windows, thermostat
3. Positioning	Adjust hospital bed	Use pillows, other support materials to reposition
SAFETY		
1. Environment	Institution regulates lighting, water temperature, hallway use.	Nurse assesses home for possible hazards
2. Equipment	Nurse assesses for damage, sends to maintenance	Nurse assesses for damage, reports or arranges for repair
3. Medications	Nurse administers, using "five rights" as guide Nurse observes for side effects	Nurse teaches patient and family administration and side effects
COMFORT AND HYGIENE		
1. Personal Care	Type and time of care planned by nurse	Type and time of care planned by patient's wish
2. Comfort	Analgesia by doctor's order Nursing measures to promote comfort	Analgesia by doctor's order Nurse teaches comfort measures to family
ACTIVITY AND REST		
1. Ambulation	Per doctor's order, often done at nurse's convenience	Per doctor's order; done per patient's schedule
2. Sleep/Rest	Often interrupted by institutional activity	Patient sleeps as desired in familiar surroundings
NUTRITION		
1. Therapeutic diet	Per doctor's order Planned by dietitian Served on schedule Nurse reinforces diet teaching	Per doctor's order Instructions by dietitian Nurse assists in planning Nurse assesses patient's nutrition and diet plan

Table 9–2 Adapting care to meet basic needs (Continued)

NEED/ CONCERN	TRADITIONAL SETTING	PATIENT'S HOME
ELIMINATION		
1. Stool/Urine	Intake and Output records Charting of function Nurse views and notes function	Nurse interviews patient about status of kidney and bowel function
PSYCHOSOCIAL		
1. Psychological comfort	Nurse primary support Patient in strange surroundings, new people and routines	Family primary support Patient in own environment Nurse guest in home
2. Support persons	Limited visiting hours Family indirectly involved	Family present much of day Friends and neighbors more readily available for help

Health care in this country has often segregated patients in different age groups. Pediatric units are designed for children, of course, and most other units are intended for adults. Some hospitals have adolescent care units, especially for young adults with chemical dependency or mental health problems. Traditional nursing homes were designed only for elderly patients. In much of your learning, you probably may have cared for patients in only one age group at a time.

Nursing in expanded settings, however, will require that you adapt to patients of different ages. Many doctor's offices have patients ranging from newborn to the very elderly. You will need to be aware of the differing needs and concerns of these patients.

Figure 9–4 summarizes the physical changes, psychosocial stages and key health concerns of age groups.

ADDITIONAL CONCEPTS FOR ADAPTATION

Using Therapeutic Communication

Carl Rogers was a psychologist who helped shape specific therapeutic communication techniques. Therapeutic communication skills are useful when the intent of the exchange is to help the patient sort out and express his

A. 0–2 Years (Infant and Toddler)

Physical Changes

Doubles birth weight at 6 months; triples weight at 1 year
Progressive head-to-toe development

- Lifts head from prone position at one month
- Stands on toes with support at 1 year
- Walks and runs with a stiff gait at 2 years

Motor skills become more refined

- Clenches fist at 1 month
- Holds toy in hand at 6 months
- Begins fine coordination at 1 year

Psychosocial Responses

Trust vs. Mistrust; begins to identify self
Parents most important persons (mother first year)
Beginning language skills

- Smiles, coos, and makes vowel sounds by 6 months
- Has small vocabulary and imitates sounds by 1 year
- Has vocabulary of several hundred words and speaks in short sentences by 2 years

Play in social growth follows head-to-toe development

- Eyes follow colorful mobiles in crib at 1 month
- Reaches for blocks and teething toys at 6 months
- Enjoys pull/push toys at 1 year
- Builds with blocks; looks at picture books at 2 years

Key Health Concerns

- Scheduled checks with physician to monitor normal growth and development
- Infant immunizations
- Bonding with parents

Figure 9–4 Guidelines for assessment through the life span

B. 2–5 Years (Preschooler)

Physical Changes

Head-to-toe development becomes more specialized

- Begins to be independent with self-care
    Feeds self with fork; undresses self at 3 years
    Brushes teeth and dresses self at 5 years
- Motor skills develop
    Alternates feet climbing stairs at 3 years
    Has good balance and hops, skips at 5 years

Psychosocial Responses

Independent enterprise vs. Guilt
Nuclear family most important persons

- Has 900 word vocabulary; remembers and repeats three numbers at 3 years
- Asks endless questions at three; questions about word meanings at 5 years

Play and social growth

- Begins social contacts and group play at three
- Widens experiences in reading, music, and more cooperative play at five

Key Health Concerns

Continue regular physician checks to monitor growth and development; immunizations

- Promote nutrition in diet
- Teach beginning hygiene practices
- Promote healthy family interactions

Figure 9–4 (Continued)

C. 6–18 Years (Traditional school years)

Physical Changes

Growth spurts noted from 7–9 and 13–15 years

- Extremities appear longer in proportion to body
- Beginning secondary sex characteristics at 9–11 for girls, 11–13 for boys
    Menstruation onset 11–14 years
    Capable of reproduction

Motor skills continue to develop

- More coordinated; fine hand movements at 8 years
- More physically active by 12 years
- Increased muscular ability and coordination—12–18 years

Psychosocial Response

Industry vs. Inferiority 6–12 years

- Neighbor and school friends most important persons

Identity vs. Role Confusion 12–18 years

- Peer, organizational groups most important persons

Play and social development

- Group play with own sex 6–12 years
    Dramatic play: school, wants to be fireman at 7
    Board, card games, books, music at 10
    School sports, clubs at 12
- More heterosexual group activity 12–18 years
    Learns to be more self-sufficient

Key Health Concerns

Provide safety education

- Crossing street, riding bike, driving car

Figure 9–4 (Continued)

Promote healthy lifestyle

- Provide education in health issues: nutrition, drugs, smoking, alcohol, sexual behavior

Promote healthy interactions with family, peers

D. 19–40 Years (Young and Middle Adulthood)

Physical Changes

Complete physical and sexual development
Beginning signs of aging process; graying, hair thinning, "crows feet"
Motor skills continue to develop

- Activity vs. inactivity with each individual
- Influences: job, interest areas

Psychosocial Responses

Intimacy vs. Isolation
Friends and sexual partners most important persons

- Forms lasting relationships with others

Focus on beginning family and job responsibilities

Key Health Concerns

Promote healthy lifestyle to avoid health risks: obesity, diabetes, heart disease, hypertension
Encourage prenatal care for all pregnant women

E. 40–65 Years (Middle and Later Adulthood)

Physical Changes

Visible signs of aging process in all individuals
Influences: heredity, job, lifestyle, health practices
Motor skills continue healthy influence: activity vs. inactivity

Figure 9–4 (Continued)

Psychosocial Response

Creative, active vs. Stagnation

- Productive, creative, relaxed competitiveness
    May be the most productive years of life
- Stagnation results from refusal to be responsible for goals of middle age

Family of several generations very important

- Assists next generation to be responsible adults

Key Health Concerns

Promote healthy lifestyle

- Focus includes nutrition, exercise, reduced stress

Encourage annual physician visit to monitor early warning signs of disease

- Additional diagnostic studies for risk groups:
    Pap smear, mammogram–women
    Chest x-ray, sputum specimen–smokers
    Proctoscope—>40, family history cancer
    Blood work, stress EKG—obese, >risk CVD

Promote healthy family, job, community interactions

- Community support groups available

F. 65 + (65–75 Young Old; 75–85 Old; 85–Old Old)

Physical Changes

All body functions slowed with aging process
- Rate of change affected by life-style of life span
- Motor skills continue at slower pace
    Tasks remain accurate; influenced only by time

Figure 9–4 (Continued)

Psychosocial Response

Ego integrity vs. Despair

- Satisfied with life as meaningful, continues on
- Despair results from feelings of failure and that it is too late to change

Adjustments to life after retirement
Adjustments to loss of spouse; faces death as daily part of life with loss of friends, relatives
Increasing dependency (particularly after 85)
Loneliness

Key Health Concerns

Maintain function and maximum independence
Monitor life span and aging health risks of individual
Adequate income to afford medical care
Family and social interactions to promote self-worth

Figure 9–4 (Continued)

KEY CONCEPT: REVIEW OF SOME CONCEPTS TO ADAPT

- The Nursing Process includes making assessments to develop a nursing diagnosis, planning, implementing, and evaluating the care.
- Maslow's Theory of Basic Needs focuses on meeting physiological survival needs before addressing psychosocial needs.
- Erikson's Theory of Ages and Stages explains developmental changes throughout the life span.

UNIT 9/ADAPTING BASIC NURSING CONCEPTS TO EXPANDED SETTINGS

feelings. You have probably learned many of these skills in your nursing education.

Using open-ended statements and listening intently, without being judgmental, are two examples of therapeutic communication skills. Reflecting what the patient says is another example.

There are also some identifiable blocks to successful communication. When you inadvertently use a cliché, you sometimes interfere with meaningful conversation with a patient. See figure 9–5 for a review of techniques that are helpful and some that may be detrimental.

Identifying Cultural Differences and Family Systems

In Section Two you learned how the community, culture, and family affect the patient. Again, it is important to remember that every patient is part of a greater picture. The person you meet belongs to a family and a community. His reaction to you, as well as yours to him, is greatly influenced by those other relationships.

When you are nursing in expanded settings you will become acutely aware of the cultural differences between patients. In the hospital, everyone looks alike; hospital gowns and beds are not very individualized. But when you see a patient in his home, you will realize that this is a unique individual who likes classical music, or hard rock, or paints pictures as a hobby, or collects stamps.

The patient's family also gains importance in the expanded care setting. The adolescent diabetic in the hospital may appear confident about managing diet and insulin. When she returns to the clinic with her mother she may be timid and shy; mom does all the talking and complaining. How will you deal with this?

Assisting with Patient Teaching

Every aspect of nursing and patient care involves patient teaching. You have done this many times informally as you helped patients recover from acute conditions. Perhaps you have encouraged a postoperative patient to walk, by explaining the importance of re-establishing peristalsis. You have also done patient teaching when you encouraged long term care residents to maintain a level of function. The emphasis is just as important when you encourage the nursing home patient to walk so as to maintain function of his arthritic joints. Knowledge, attitudes, and skills are as vital to patients' education as they are to nurses' education!

Patient education continues to be important in expanded settings. Nurses may not be available "round the clock" to answer questions and

DO:

Use broad opening statements.
    "Is there something bothering you?"
    "Would you like to talk about it?"

Use general leads.
    "Oh?"
    "Ummm...."

Acknowledge patient's thoughts.
    "You wonder if it's helping...."
    "You're upset because...."

Share your observations with the patient.
    "You appear angry."
    "You seem quite calm at the moment."

Give information.
    "The dietitian said...."
    "The van will pick you up at 11 A.M."

DON'T:

Disagree
    "That's not what she meant."
    "You're wrong."

Use social clichés.
    "Everything will be just fine!"
    "Did you hear the story about...."

Assume you've solved the problem.
    "There, now you're feeling better."
    "That takes care of it, then."

Figure 9–5 DOs and DON'Ts of therapeutic communication

monitor patient progress. Therefore, plans for patient teaching are completed in a variety of ways in clinics, home health care, and other settings. In physicians' offices, patients may be given informational booklets for procedures scheduled in surgical centers. Figures 9–6 and 9–7 are examples of instructional information given to patients. The pre-exam/surgery teaching is reinforced by the surgical center nurses, figure 9–8.

In home health care, the patient teaching format may be quite similar to those in hospitals and long term care facilities. These plans are developed by the case coordinator and the community health team. As the nurse involved, you will be delegated specific steps in the teaching plan or expected to provide reinforcement of earlier teaching. Your broader role may be that of keen observer and data collector.

It will be helpful for you to understand basic guidelines in planning patient teaching. These will assist you in reporting data on patient readiness and response to learning.

Know Your Patient. To be effective in patient teaching, you must first start by assessing the patient accurately. What is he or she like? What is his or her knowledge level regarding the condition? Are there any special learning needs, such as language problems or hearing deficits? If special needs exist, planning the patient teaching may require modification.

Next, you need to know the patient's interests. What does he or she *want* to know about the condition? Third, you are one of the experts, so you must decide what the patient *needs* to know. There is much information available, but you should limit yourself to what the patient really needs to understand in order to contribute to the recovery.

Mr. Schmidt, a 55-year old farmer, had an abdomino-perineal resection for rectal cancer. When discharged from the hospital, he apparently understood how to irrigate his colostomy. As the home health nurse, you are supposed to observe the irrigation procedure. After you get acquainted, you ask him how he is managing the irrigations at home. He responds by saying he hasn't tried it yet because he's waiting for his bowels to move "the regular way." It is obvious that Mr. Schmidt will need more teaching than you were led to believe! His knowledge level about his condition is nearly zero. Since he has been home for two days, and eating quite well, he needs to have an irrigation today. Where can you begin? It may be helpful to sketch a picture of the intestines, review their function, and explain to him that he now has a new way to evacuate waste. He may be familiar with elimination problems that farm animals develop. Then you could explain that you will help him with today's irrigation. That may be all you can accomplish on this visit.

Plan the Teaching. The nurse and the patient should discuss the teaching goals and plan them together whenever possible. Objectives should be given

```
Ophthalmology                                          Telephone (612) 437-2060
Ophthalmic Surgery

                    DAVID A. HENDRICKSON, M.D., P.A.
                       204 REGINA MEDICAL CENTER
                       HASTINGS, MINNESOTA 55033


    OUTPATIENT CATARACT SURGERY PRE-OPERATIVE INSTRUCTIONS    DATE_____
    TO: _____

    1. YOUR CATARACT SURGERY IS SCHEDULED FOR _____.
    2. THE ANESTHESIA TO BE USED IS _____,
    3. PLEASE DO NOT EAT OR DRINK ANYTHING AFTER MIDNIGHT _____.
    4. TAKE YOUR REGULAR MEDICINES AS USUAL THE MORNING OF SURGERY. YOU MAY DRINK
       WATER TO SWALLOW YOUR MEDICINES.
    5. PLEASE REPORT TO THE ADMISSIONS OFFICE AT _____
       _____ AT _____ A.M. ON _____.
    6. THE NIGHT BEFORE SURGERY PLEASE REMOVE ALL FACIAL MAKE-UP, PERFUMES, ETC. WASH
       YOUR FACE WITH SOAP AND WATER.
    7. DO NOT APPLY ANY FACIAL MAKE-UP OF FACIAL POWDERS ON THE MORNING OF SURGERY.
    8. PLEASE PUT TOBREX DROPS IN YOUR _____ EYE FOUR TIMES A DAY STARTING
       _____.
    9. A PRESCRIPTION FOR THE TOBREX DROPS IS ENCLOSED. YOU MAY HAVE THIS PRESCRIPTION
       FILLED AT ANY PHARMACY.
    10. ENCLOSED ARE TWO FORMS: (A) A MEDICAL HISTORY QUESTIONNAIRE AND (B) AN INFORMED
        CONSENT. PLEASE REVIEW AND COMPLETE AND SIGN THESE FORMS. BRING THE FORMS TO
        THE HOSPITAL THE DAY OF SURGERY.
    11. A SHORT FORM HISTORY & PHYSICAL FORM IS ALSO ENCLOSED. PLEASE MAKE AN
        APPOINTMENT TO SEE YOUR REGULAR MEDICAL DOCTOR FOR A BRIEF PRE-OPERATIVE CHECK-UP
        PRIOR TO THE DAY OF SURGERY. (BRING THIS COMPLETED FORM TO THE HOSPITAL.)
    11. IF YOU HAVE ANY QUESTIONS, OR SOMETHING IS NOT CLEAR, PLEASE CALL THE OFFICE
        AT 437-2060. (AREA CODE 612).
```

Figure 9–6 Sample outpatient preoperative instructions (Courtesy of David A. Hendrickson, M.D.)

UNIT 9/ADAPTING BASIC NURSING CONCEPTS TO EXPANDED SETTINGS

Ophthalmology
Ophthalmic Surgery

Telephone (612) 437-2060

DAVID A. HENDRICKSON, M.D., P.A.
204 REGINA MEDICAL CENTER
HASTINGS, MINNESOTA 55033

POST-OPERATIVE CATARACT SURGERY INSTRUCTIONS

1. YOU MAY RESUME YOUR USUAL ROUTINE ACTIVITIES.
2. AVOID EXCESSIVE STRAINING, COUGHING OR HEAVY LIFTING.
3. YOU MAY READ, WRITE, WATCH TELEVISION AS YOU DESIRE.
4. YOUR EYES MAY WATER. AVOID RUBBING THEM.
5. WEAR YOUR GLASSES DURING THE DAY.
6. WEAR DARK GLASSES WHEN OUT OF DOORS. YOUR EYE WILL BE SENSITIVE TO LIGHT.
7. SLEEP WITH YOUR EYE SHIELD TAPED IN PLACE OVER YOUR EYE. IF POSSIBLE, SLEEP ON YOUR BACK OR YOUR UNOPERATED SIDE.
8. INSTRUCTIONS FOR THE USE OF YOUR EYEDROPS WILL BE GIVEN AT YOUR FIRST POST-OPERATIVE VISIT.
9. TO PUT IN YOUR EYEDROPS, PLACE THE INDEX FINGER ON YOUR CHEEKBONE, PULLING THE LOWER LID DOWN. LOOK UP. HAVE THE MEDICINE DROPPED INSIDE THE LOWER LID.
10. BRING ALL YOUR EYEDROPS TO YOUR POST-OPERATIVE OFFICE VISITS.
11. USE YOUR MEDICINES AS DIRECTED:
    A. _____
    B. _____
12. IF AT ANY TIME YOU HAVE A SHARP OR CONTINUOUS PAIN IN YOUR EYE, PLEASE CALL THE OFFICE.
13. YOUR FIRST POST-OPERATIVE VISIT IS SCHEDULED FOR _____
    AT _____.
    PLEASE LEAVE THE PATCH AND SHIELD IN PLACE UNTIL SEEN IN THE OFFICE.
14. IF YOU ARE NOT ABLE TO KEEP THE ABOVE APPOINTMENT, PLEASE CALL THE OFFICE AT 437-2060. (AREA CODE 612)

Figure 9–7 Sample outpatient postoperative instructions (Courtesy of David A. Hendrickson, M.D.)

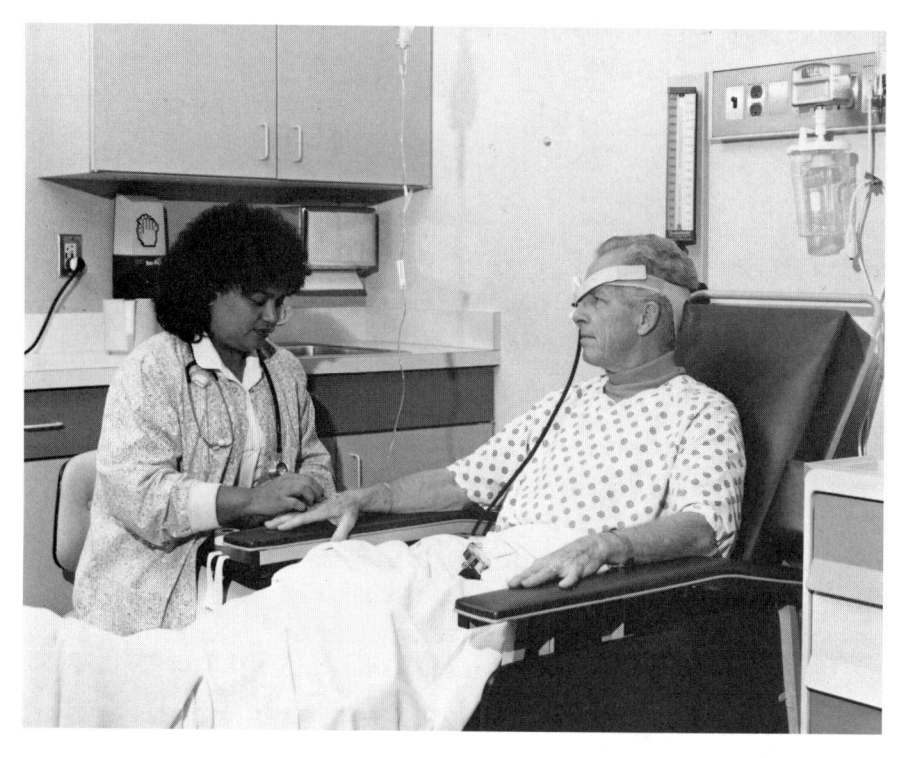

Figure 9–8 During preoperative care, the surgi-center nurse reinforces patient teaching before cataract surgery.

in clear, simple terms, and reflect realistic goals. They should be measurable; that is, you want to see some definite results.

Mr. Schmidt's situation should be discussed with the case coordinator. Perhaps the coordinator will make a home visit to help plan the teaching. You may be asked by the coordinator to return and continue reviewing the colostomy irrigation procedure.

On your next visit, you may ask Mr. Schmidt to review what he had learned about his condition from the doctor and the hospital nurses. Then you can build on that information to reinforce the importance of continuing irrigations every two days until the bowel becomes regulated. The goals he could set with you might include his being able to do the procedure independently.

Special Notes to Nurses. It is important to remember some basic communication rules when involved with patient teaching. Accept the patient where he is. Offer praise. Be sensitive to the patient's individuality. Be alert for teaching opportunities. These basic principles of patient education are summarized in figure 9–9.

Patient Learning and Trauma. Jane M. Lee developed a theory about reactions to trauma, stating that four distinct stages exist. The first stage is *impact*, which is the initial reaction. It often includes fear of loss or of death. The next stage is *regression*, which includes denial, and the fear of not being loved.

The third stage is called *acknowledgment*, when the person mourns and suffers a loss of self-esteem. The last stage is *reconstruction*, and happens when the person is ready to get on with his life.

This theory has been combined with Maslow's hierarchy of needs to help explain why patient teaching is not always successful. The person in the impact stage cannot begin to understand what is being presented. Learning is most effective in the reconstruction stage.

- KNOW THE PATIENT

    What is the knowledge level?
    What is the interest level?
    Is the patient emotionally ready to learn?
    Are there any special factors to consider in planning?

- KNOW THE SUBJECT

    Review the condition.
    Has there been a change in body function?
    What does the patient need to know?

- PLAN THE TEACHING/LEARNING GOALS

    Include the patient.
    Establish realistic goals.
    Goals should be measurable.

Figure 9–9 Principles of patient teaching

Because patients leave hospitals quickly, it is often nurses in expanded care settings who will complete the necessary patient teaching. The meshing of Lee's theory with Maslow's theory and suggestions for patient education is illustrated in figure 9–10. During the impact stage, the person's physiological and safety needs are threatened. At this point the patient must be protected. Questions should be answered, but no in-depth teaching should be attempted. The patient needs explanations, support, and someone to listen.

Regression affects social needs. The patient needs to know that you accept him and think well of him. Necessary instructions should be simple. In this stage, it is necessary to establish rapport.

Acknowledgment relates to the person's esteem needs. The patient is ready to be more active in the learning process. He may ask more questions. The stage of reconstruction meshes with Maslow's self-actualization concept. Now the patient is ready to plan ahead. The nurse may be a referral person at this point.

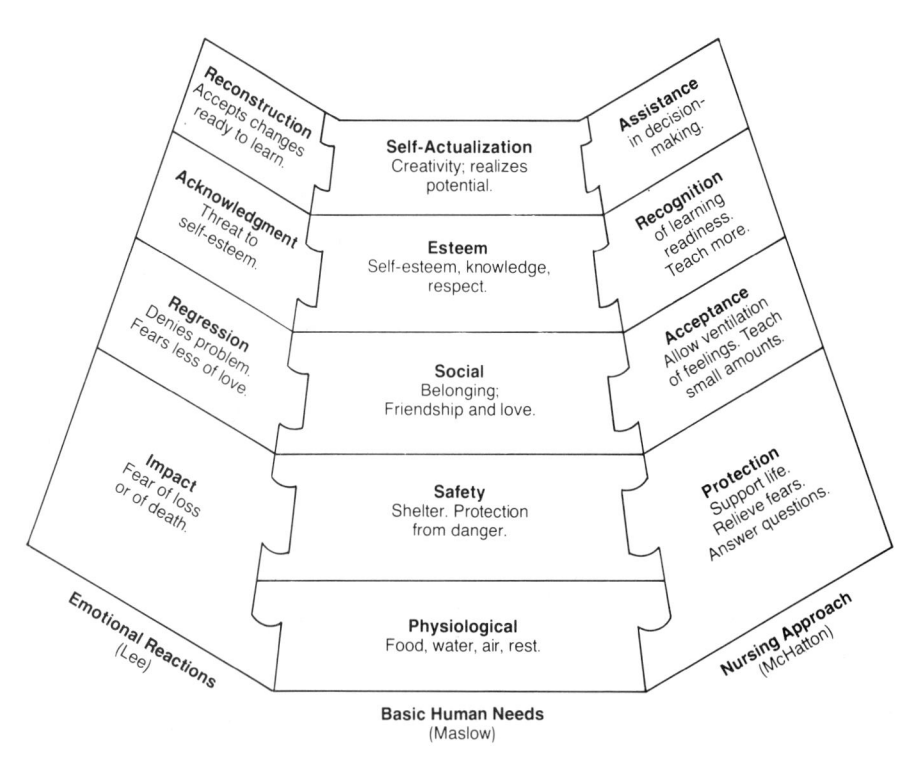

Figure 9–10 Readiness to learn after trauma (Adapted, with permission, from *American Journal of Nursing*, July, Vol. 85, No. 7. Copyright 1985 by American Journal of Nursing Company. "A Theory of Timely Teaching" by Maureen McHatton)

UNIT 9/ADAPTING BASIC NURSING CONCEPTS TO EXPANDED SETTINGS

> ### *KEY CONCEPT: MORE CONCEPTS TO REVIEW*
>
> - Communication skills are important nursing tools.
> - Understanding differences among cultures and families are important nursing tools.
> - Principles of teaching and learning apply to all nursing care.

Sample Patient Situation

Mrs. Viola Simpson, age 70, was dismissed from the hospital three days ago following surgery for rectal cancer. She has lived alone for five years since her husband died. A daughter lives in the same community. Before leaving the hospital, Mrs. Simpson received instructions on irrigating her colostomy with 500 milliliters of Normal Saline. Her doctor has ordered this procedure twice a week to assist in regulating bowel function.

Using the steps of the nursing process, compare and contrast the nurse's role in assisting Mrs. Simpson with her irrigation. First, identify the steps the nurse often follows in the hospital, then try to do the same as the home health nurse, using table 9–3 as a guide.

Table 9–3 Comparison of hospital and home procedures for a colostomy irrigation

HOSPITAL	HOME
ASSESSMENT	

1. Objective Data:
   a. chart: doctor's order, previous nurses' notes for irrigation results
   b. kardex: see treatment list for times of irrigation
	1. Objective Data:
	   a. care plan done by case coordinator at time of discharge
	   b. floor plan: bathroom arrangements
	      1) room for 2 people?
	      2) door hook for bag?
	      3) space for supplies?

2. Subjective Data:
   a. verify previous irrigation with the patient
      1) how did it go?
      2) did you help?
      3) any questions?
	2. Subjective Data:
	   a. interview the patient and the daughter
	      1) investigate their feelings about hospital irrigation
	      2) establish knowledge base
	      3) how much have they done?

Table 9–3 Comparison of hospital and home procedures for a colostomy irrigation (Continued)

HOSPITAL	HOME
3. Rationale: to establish the patient's level of understanding and ability to assist with procedure.	3. Rationale: to establish their level of understanding and ability to assist; to determine effectiveness of irrigation to promote bowel function; to determine the daughter's ability to assist and support.

PLANNING

1. Prepare equipment
   a. check unit for supplies (if none, send request to CSR)
   b. obtain IV pole
   c. obtain normal saline from cart
	1. Prepare equipment
	   a. assist patient in assembling equipment (brought home from hospital)
	   b. instruct the patient in preparing saline: 1 teaspoon of salt in 1 pint water
	   c. ask the patient to explain each step

2. Prepare the patient and unit
   a. make sure bathroom is available
   b. instruct the patient about the procedure
   c. instruct the patient on her participation
	2. Prepare the patient's bathroom
	   a. assist the patient in planning placement of supplies

IMPLEMENTATION

1. Complete the procedure in the patient's bathroom (if the patient is weak, do the procedure with her in bed, using an irrigation bag in bedpan)	1. Observe the patient's complete irrigation 2. Assist and support as needed 3. Praise efforts

EVALUATION

1. Determine how the patient tolerated procedure 2. Examine results	1. Determine the patient's confidence and ability 2. Assist the patient in examining results 3. Determine the need for aid and support from the daughter 4. Determine the need for a nurse to continue as a coach and support person

UNIT 9/ADAPTING BASIC NURSING CONCEPTS TO EXPANDED SETTINGS

SUMMARY

Several ideas common to nursing education have been reviewed. The nursing process and the theory of basic needs are helpful tools to use when observing patients and collecting data, whatever the setting. Recognizing that patients' concerns and attitudes are different at various ages in their lives is also helpful knowledge. Communication skills improve with practice and experience throughout life.

Identifying family and cultural differences contribute to holistic care. Helping patients to learn includes understanding their readiness to learn. When you practice nursing in expanded settings, you will be more autonomous than you have been in traditional settings. The amount of freedom you have will depend on the setting and the patients.

FOR DISCUSSION

- Collect data about the basic needs of one of your patients. Which need is most important? How would the care plan be changed if the patient were at home?

- Arrange a skit with a classmate to demonstrate therapeutic communication. Identify the techniques used.

- Develop a teaching plan for a seven-year-old boy who is going home in a spica cast.

- Patient situation: Sean Ryan, age 26, has a spinal cord injury due to a motorcycle accident six weeks ago. He is paralyzed from L-4. He has been receiving daily physical therapy while hospitalized. His goal is to return to living as independently as possible. Sean and his brother Pat are partners in a motorcycle repair shop. Pat and his wife live in the same apartment complex as Sean. Part of Sean's nursing care has included passive range-of-motion exercises of his lower extremities and active range-of-motion exercises of his upper extremities t.i.d. Use the steps in the nursing process to compare and contrast the nurse's role in carrying out this activity as (1) the nurse in the hospital, and (2) as the home health care nurse. Use table 9–3 as a guide.

QUESTIONS FOR REVIEW

1. List the components of the Nursing Process.

2. Arrange these needs in their correct priority according to Maslow's theory: oxygen, food, self-actualization, safety, spirituality, sex, belonging to a group.

3. What are three health concerns of infants and toddlers?
4. What are three health concerns of young adults?
5. List four rules for establishing therapeutic communication with a patient.
6. How does the patient's family affect health care?
7. Give one important guideline for patient education.

10
Applying Basic Concepts to Practice in Expanded Settings

OBJECTIVES:

After completing this unit, you will be able to:

- Develop a care plan for a patient receiving home health care.
- Develop a care plan for a patient seen regularly in a clinic or doctor's office.
- Adapt a teaching plan for an adult with a short attention span.
- Simulate telephone data-collection skills.
- List responsibilities of the nurse working in clinics, ambulatory surgery units, home health care, and other expanded settings.

In the preceding unit, we reviewed some of the basic concepts used in nursing education. This unit will illustrate application of these ideas in several of the expanded settings.

WORKING IN A CLINIC OR OFFICE SETTING

Working in a clinic with many doctors and/or nurse practitioners is attractive to most nurses. Working hours may be more convenient than those in a hospital; however, future clinics may need nurses working 24 hours per day. In clinics or offices, the nurse is usually working under the direction of the physician.

There is also a challenge presented by seeing many patients with assorted problems. The medical office or clinic really needs a nurse generalist; a variety of nursing skills are performed in this setting. One day you may assist with a cast application, set up several sterile fields, weigh and measure an infant, remove sutures, administer medications, and take 35 blood pressures. This is done in addition to screening telephone calls for the physician, interviewing new patients, sterilizing instruments, and preparing examination rooms!

Large clinics usually employ other workers as well as nurses. Some of these may include: receptionists, bookkeepers, laboratory and x-ray technicians, medical secretaries, and an office manager. In these settings, the nurse will probably be involved in preparing examination rooms; greeting and screening patients; assisting the doctor with specific treatments, such as Pap smears or suturing; and keeping records.

In many geographic areas, offices have only one or two doctors in practice. These physicians expect the nurses they employ to perform some clerical and minor laboratory functions as well as assist them with patients. If you already possess some clerical skills from previous employment you may find those skills useful. Keyboarding for the computer is one example of a skill that is useful in a variety of employment settings.

Sometimes a doctor in an independent practice will teach the nurse routine laboratory procedures such as checking hemoglobins. Taking an electrocardiograph (ECG) or taking an x-ray of an extremity are other procedures that you may learn on the job.

Greeting and screening patients for the doctor or nurse specialist will require conscientious use of observation skills. It is also important to observe the nonverbal responses of the patient. You will probably weigh patients, measure vital signs, and conduct a brief interview. If this is a new patient, you may be expected to collect data related to the health history. The patient is also instructed to prepare for the doctor's examination by undressing and putting on the exam gown. Some patients may need help with this.

Assisting the physician with specific procedures, such as wound suturing, will require competency in sterile techniques. With pediatric patients, it may be necessary to recall normal growth and development in order to relate effectively. You must always observe, listen, and be helpful to all patients.

Identifying a priority situation is an important responsibility. Emergencies can occur in clinic settings, or patients may come to the clinic from an accident, or with early symptoms of myocardial infarction. A patient may have an anaphylactic reaction to an allergy injection. You must keep First Aid and CPR skills current. Checking the equipment and emergency supplies is another responsibility.

UNIT 10/APPLYING BASIC CONCEPTS TO PRACTICE IN EXPANDED SETTINGS

Office nurses are also involved in patient teaching. Figure 10–1 illustrates a nurse explaining care of a cast. The doctor may give the patient a pamphlet or some information, figure 10–2. The nurse may need to clarify or simplify the information for the patient. Explaining the use of medication for its best effect is a common example. Perhaps the doctor has prescribed Lasix, 20 milligrams orally, once daily. The patient may need to be told that it should be taken in the morning instead of bedtime because Lasix increases urination for several hours and would disturb sleep.

When working in a doctor's office, you will learn how much patient education the doctor does and how much is delegated to you. A patient who is scheduled for Ambulatory Care Surgery, for example, requires specific details. What is the arrival time? Should he bring a urine specimen? Can food and fluids be taken before the procedure or not? How long will he have to stay? Can he drive home after the surgery? Should the usual medications be taken that day? Refer to clinic protocols.

Telephone triage is another common function of the office nurse. Patients often call the office with questions that may or may not need the doctor's attention. It is your job to determine which calls require a medical

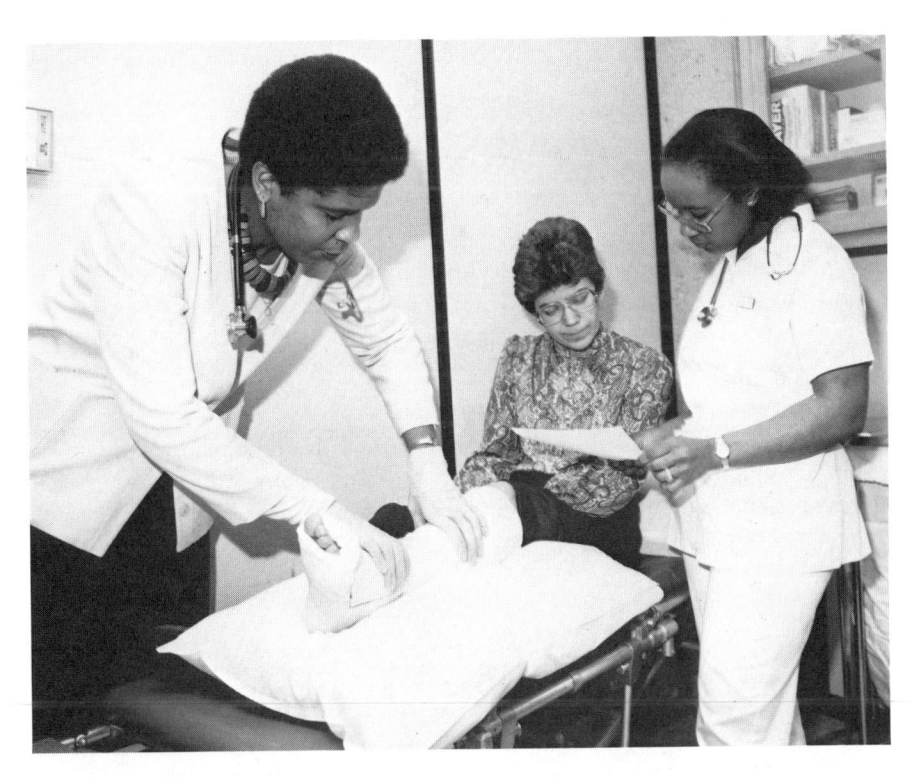

Figure 10–1 Clinic nurse explains how to protect a cast at home.

PATIENT INFORMATION

INSTRUCTIONS FOR HOME CAST CARE

The cast is a valuable piece of equipment with a specific purpose. Keep it clean and dry.

- DO NOT wash the cast or allow it to get wet.
- DO NOT walk on wet surfaces or grass at anytime.
- DO NOT walk on the cast unless the doctor applied a walking heel or a cast boot and has given permission to do so.
- DO NOT use any instrument to scratch under the cast. Some itching under the cast is to be expected.
- DO NOT put anything under the cast (pennies and other objects cause bad pressure sores).
- DO NOT use talcum or baby powder on the skin around the cast or between the toes. Use alcohol on a Q-tip or a small piece of cotton to clean between toes and around the cast.

Complications do occur under a cast. Early recognition is very important. Please watch for and report the following:

- Pain under the cast.
- Numbness and tingling of fingers or toes.
- Swelling of toes and fingers.
- Any change in color or temperature of feet or hands. They should feel warm and color should be pink.
- Any discharge or strange odor or staining on/or under the cast.
- Breaking or softening of the cast.

The first four can often be avoided by elevating the arm or leg on a pillow so the extremity is higher than the chest. Contact the clinic if any of these symptoms persist after attempting elevation on a pillow.

Additional Instructions:

Figure 10–2 Patient instructions for home cast care

opinion and refer them to the doctor. This means that you should develop good telephone interviewing skills. (This is also called *data collection.*) You should know what kinds of questions to ask, depending on the patient's condition and what you already know about the caller. Keep a medication reference book near the phone so that you can easily refer to it about medication actions and side effects. Basic telephone etiquette for a health care setting is reviewed in figure 10–3.

Keeping the records up to date is another responsibility. Each clinic or office will have its own routine forms and procedures. Accuracy and thoroughness is vital. Continuity of care requires complete documentation. Accuracy is also necessary for proper reimbursement by third party payers.

BE PREPARED! Have drug references, memo pads, pencils near the phone. Have the patient's chart available when returning a call.

PUT ON A SMILE! Smiling projects acceptance. Speak clearly into the mouthpiece. Identify yourself. Project a caring attitude.

PROJECT PROFESSIONAL PRESENCE! Use correct grammer. Concentrate on the caller, not side-discussions with others. Use technical terms when appropriate. Avoid slang.

SCREEN CALLS TACTFULLY! Employers will help you learn which calls will need their attention. Some patients prefer speaking with the doctor. Your knowledge base about signs and symptoms, medications and side effects is very important.

COLLECT DATA THOROUGHLY! Who is calling? Why? Who is the patient? What is the problem? Ask specific questions related to the system involved and the symptoms.

GIVE INFORMATION CLEARLY! Be clear and concise. Ask callers if they understand the given information.

USE HOLD CAUTIOUSLY! Ask the caller to wait before using hold; be sure it is not an emergency call.

CLOSE POLITELY! Summarize the decision or action to be taken. Explain when you will return the call or have an answer. Let the caller hang up first.

Figure 10–3 Basic telephone etiquette

Various kinds of payment plans were described in Unit 3. You should be acquainted with the plans available in your community so that you can answer questions whenever necessary and know what should be referred to another resource. There may be referrals made to other health care providers; when you are aware of the resources you can guide the patient to the best choice.

KEY CONCEPT: RESPONSIBILITIES OF OFFICE NURSES

- Patient screening
- Patient interviews, in person and by telephone
- Identifying priority situations
- Assisting with specific treatments
- Patient teaching
- Preparing equipment and exam rooms
- Record keeping
- Laboratory skills

Sample Situation

Mr. Philip Goranske is a sales representative for several software vendors. His work requires frequent traveling. He has a standing appointment at the clinic to have his blood pressure checked monthly. Dr. Chaou's standing orders are that hypertensive patients with blood pressures above 160/100 should see her.

Mr. Goranske is waiting at the clinic when you arrive to unlock the door at 8:30 A.M. He says, "Check my blood pressure, will you? And please hurry, I have an 11 o'clock plane to catch." You turn on the computer, pull up his record, and note that he is a week late for his appointment. Then you weigh him and see that he has gained five pounds. His blood pressure is 156/98. He is taking hydrochlorathiazide, 50 milligrams daily.

What kind of data is available? How should you help Mr. Goranske? The doctor will be in at 9:30 A.M. What should you say to the patient?

Data: Busy man, appears stressed
Did appear, even if late
Gained five pounds
Blood pressure is very near limit established by doctor

Rationale: Probably won't wait to see the doctor today
May not be taking his medication
May be careless about his diet
Visit reflects concern about health

Nursing Diagnosis: Knowledge deficit of disease/treatment

Plan: Encourage diet and medication compliance.
Tell patient your concern.
Arrange for an appointment with Dr. Chaou when Mr. Goranske will be in town.

Implementation: "I'm glad you stopped by, Mr. Goranske. Your blood pressure is 156/98, which is a little higher than it was last month. Have you been taking your pills regularly? (yes or no) I see you've also gained five pounds this month. It must be hard to follow a diet when you travel so much. It would probably be a good idea for you to see Dr. Chaou next time you're home. When will that be?"

You should then make the appointment and document this visit, including your data and impression.

Evaluation: To be done on the next visit.

WORKING IN AN AMBULATORY SURGERY CENTER

Nurses in ambulatory surgery settings can focus their caregiving on pre- and postoperative nursing. Large units may separate patients according to the kind of surgery, or keep the preoperative patients in a different area than those who are recovering.

The patient will have been given some preoperative instructions by the doctor and office nurse. It is a good plan for the ambulatory surgery nurse to telephone the patient a few days ahead of the scheduled surgery to remind him about withholding food and fluids; also, any questions he may have can be answered at this time.

When the patient arrives in the center, he will complete any forms needed for payers and sign the surgical permit. Admission nursing care may be quite brief, but you must use every opportunity to observe, educate, and reassure the patient, figure 10–4. Assessing the patient's knowledge level,

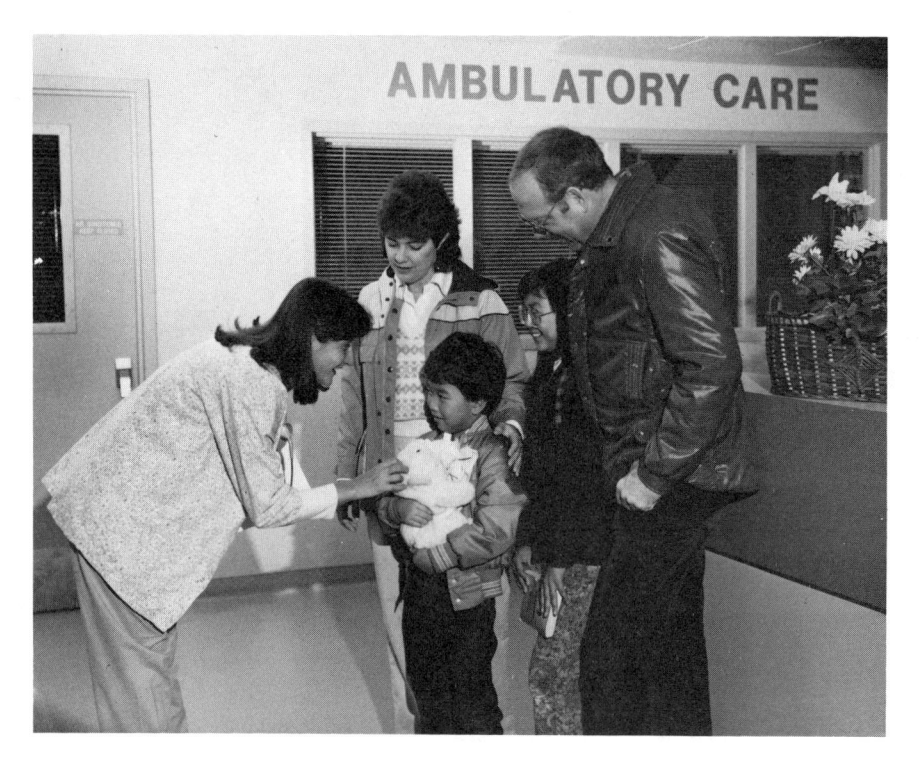

Figure 10–4 A nurse greeting a child before same-day surgery

collecting vital signs, giving prescribed medications, and answering questions will be your responsibilities.

Depending on the setting, your postoperative care may or may not include the immediate recovery period. In some settings, the patient who is given a general anesthetic may be transferred to a recovery room for the initial postoperative nursing care. Further postoperative care, such as monitoring vital signs and dressings, and noting the time of first voiding are responsibilities of the ambulatory care center. You will also be responsible for giving the patient instructions about further postoperative care to be followed at home. Most settings require that a family member or friend accompany the patient at the time of discharge; the patient may be drowsy for awhile after anesthesia. Figure 10–5 illustrates recovery care in an ambulatory surgery setting.

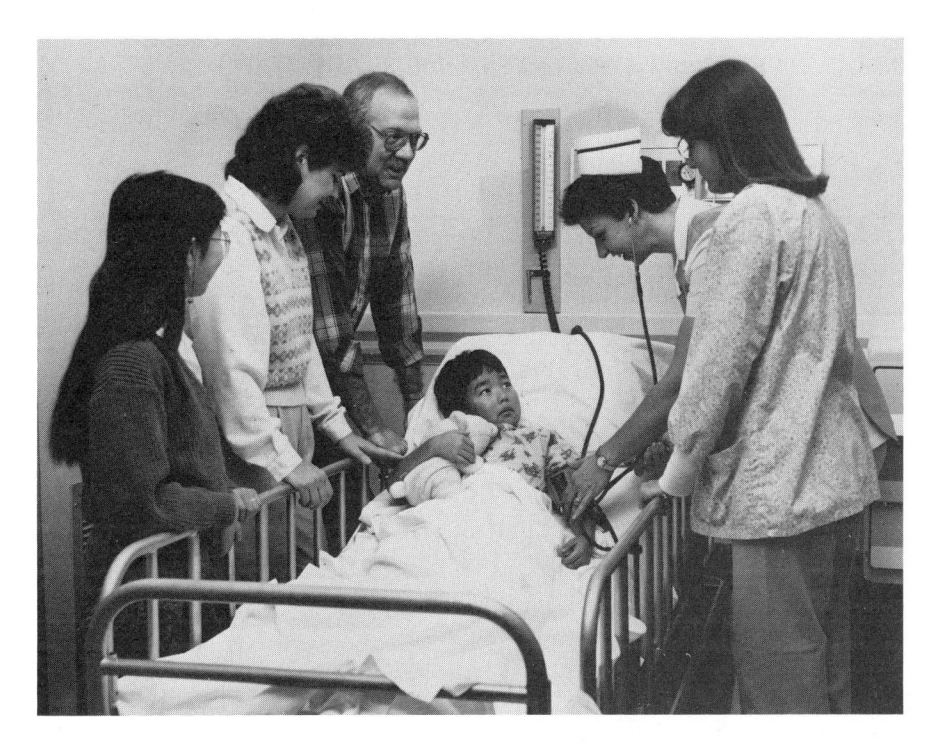

Figure 10–5 Recovery care in an ambulatory surgery setting

Patients should receive written as well as oral instructions about their self-care. Instructions should be stated simply and be concise. The patient should also have the phone numbers of the surgical center and of the doctor's office.

Within 48 hours after surgery, one of the nurses usually telephones the patient to see how he is managing. This is a good opportunity to answer any questions that may have arisen. It also promotes good public relations. Figure 10–6 shows a form used for a follow-up phone call.

Nursing practice in an ambulatory surgery setting requires good organizational skills and basic nursing knowledge. Data collection skills must be very precise because you have such a small amount of time with the patients. You may also be expected to take care of the equipment and environment.

SURGI-CENTER POST-OP TELEPHONE ASSESSMENT

A. Day of Surgery Information. (Complete before discharge.)

Name _____ Age _____ Home Phone _____

Physician _____ Date of Surgery _____

Procedure _____ Anesthesia _____

Discharge status: (surgery site, dressing, voiding, ambulation)

Discharge instructions: (physician's orders, patient teaching)

B. Home Assessment. (24–72 hours after discharge)   Date _____

Patient's general comments: (how he/she feels now, progress of recovery, eating/drinking, elimination, ambulating, meds)

Surgical site data: (drainage, pain, swelling, dressing)

Anesthesia recovery:

Patient concerns: (additional questions and concerns)

Figure 10–6 Example of surgi-center follow-up tool

UNIT 10/APPLYING BASIC CONCEPTS TO PRACTICE IN EXPANDED SETTINGS   **173**

C. Evaluation.

Review of discharge instructions:

Verify physician's office telephone number:

Further follow-up:

Nurse _____

Figure 10–6 (Continued)

KEY CONCEPT: RESPONSIBILITIES OF NURSES IN AMBULATORY SURGERY SETTINGS

- Preoperative teaching and care
- Postoperative care
- Teaching self-care for at home
- Postoperative follow-up by phone
- Documentation
- Environmental management

Sample Situation

Tua Vang, who has had chronic otitis media, is scheduled for bilateral P-E tube placement through the ambulatory surgery setting. She is 22-months old. You spoke with her mother on the telephone yesterday. She understood that Tua could not have anything to eat before coming to the surgical unit today.

PREOPERATIVE CARE PLAN

Assessment:
  Data—toddler; mother understands procedure.
  Rationale—will need parent near much of time; little pre-op physical care will be needed.

Nursing Diagnosis: Fear related to an unfamiliar environment.

Plan: Try to gain child's trust. Have parent undress her and put on surgery gown. Complete paperwork for surgery.

Implementation: Calmly and politely offer any explanations. Carry out plan.

Evaluation: Is the child ready for surgery?

POSTOPERATIVE CARE PLAN

Assessment:
  Data—cries whenever awakened. Pulse 106 at rest, respirations 28. Pink nailbeds, conjunctiva, and oral mucosa. No drainage from either ear.
  Rationale—Seems stable at present time.

Nursing Diagnosis: Comfort, alteration in, pain.

Plan: Reassure parent, allow her to be with child. Continue monitoring vital signs according to policy. Review discharge instructions with parent.

Implementation: Carry out plan.

Evaluation: Is the child stable and ready to be discharged? Is the parent comfortable about continuing the care?

WORKING IN A HOME HEALTH CARE SETTING

Home health care agencies are experiencing rapid growth as part of the health care delivery system. Employment with such an agency can offer flexible hours, regular work, a variety of patients, and the satisfaction many nurses find in spending concentrated time with only one patient at a time. A generalist with a broad basic knowledge of nursing and human behavior is best suited for this work. Also, it will be necessary to function autonomously. Some agencies prefer that nurses have at least one year of hospital experience before seeking employment in home health care.

It is the case coordinator's responsibility to make the initial visit to the patient, at home or in the hospital, in order to do a total assessment interview. A sample tool for home health care assessment can be found in Appendix B. The physician's orders, the patient's needs and the type of payment plan will then help determine assignments for nurses, aides, homemakers or other types of caregivers. The case coordinator will assign you according to the patient's care plan.

The case coordinator may schedule your visit with the patient or you may be expected to do that yourself. Review the initial assessment and care plan before your visit. Allow some extra time to find the home on your first visit, unless you know the area very well. Remember that you are a guest in the patient's home. Do not judge the patient or family by the type of housing, part of town, or how they keep house. Your values of orderliness or cleanliness may be different than theirs, but it is their home. As long as the patient is safe, you must not interfere.

On the first visit, you may want to spend some time getting acquainted with the patient and whatever family is present. They will want to know a little bit about you, too. You can tell them how long you've been a nurse, for example, and why you enjoy home health care. You need not share your total life. Establishing their trust in you is very important. They will cooperate and follow your suggestions more closely if they feel you are competent and trustworthy. While you are visiting, you should be making mental observations about the environment and the family's interactions. Review Unit 8 for family assessment skills. Suggested steps in making a home health care visit are given in figure 10-7.

The visit may be scheduled for only 30 minutes or up to eight hours, depending on the care you are assigned to give. Try to stay within the time allotted. Carry out your responsibilities efficiently. Perhaps you are to do range of motion exercises on a paralyzed extremity. First, help the patient into a comfortable position. Be sure he understands what you are going to do and the reason for the treatment. Then go through the exercises slowly and smoothly, watching for nonverbal responses as well as listening to comments or complaints.

Sometimes it might be necessary to improvise equipment in the home. A small washtub may be used as for a foot soak. You should know how to convert metric numbers to household measurements. The young mother giving medication may not know that 15 milliliters or cc's is the same as a measured tablespoon. Normal saline can be made with one pint of water and one teaspoon of table salt.

Some equipment, such as bedside commodes or walkers, is readily available through medical supply companies or the local drugstore. Organizations, such as the American Cancer Society, may also provide special equipment for patients.

1. Receive assignment.
2. Contact patient or caregiver to schedule visit.
3. Review assessment and nursing care plan.
4. Arrive at patient's home at planned time.
5. Introduce self. Short get-acquainted chat. Be attentive to environment and non-verbal communication.
6. Deliver needed supplies and equipment.
7. Give care and reinforce teaching as needed.
8. Collect data about patient, family, health condition, environment.
9. Close visit as appropriate.
10. Complete documentation.
11. Report to case coordinator.

Figure 10–7 Steps in making a home health visit

When your visit is over, complete whatever documentation is required by the agency. This may include nurses' notes as well as other records. Also, keep your own record of travel costs. Whether your employer pays you for traveling or not, the records may be helpful for your tax files.

Reporting to the case coordinator may take place as often as needed. Many agencies have regular, scheduled, care planning meetings. Sometimes it is permissible to report by phone or by mail. Be sure that the case coordinator is aware of changes observed in the patient or the home situation.

You should be aware of payment plans used by patients served through your agency. Knowledge about the kinds of records and documentation required are very important for reimbursement by government or private insurers. As with all charting, "If it isn't documented, it wasn't done." This means that the cost of dressings or other supplies won't be reimbursed by a third-party payer if the nurses' records don't show that they were needed and used. See figure 10–8 for sample records.

Home health care nurses must be able to tell when the patient and family can manage without help. If you are successful in your care, they won't need you anymore! It is not advisable to give patients your home phone number. This is to prevent the patient from becoming too dependent and to keep you from becoming too involved. It is easy to feel like a member of the family if you are with them through difficult times or for several

UNIT 10/APPLYING BASIC CONCEPTS TO PRACTICE IN EXPANDED SETTINGS 177

DOB 11/7/15
married

SHAMROCK IN-HOME NURSING CARE, INC.

Date of Admission 12/18/86 _____ phone 281-3538
PATIENT'S NAME John Smith _____ Address 106 Maple St. Rochester, MN 55901
Religion Lutheran _____ Drug Allergies NKA
Age 71 Height 5'9" Weight 62.2 Diet 90 meq sodium
Hearing good Vision glasses Speech clear Dental upper and lower dentures
Diagnosis Congestive heart failure, history of pulmonary edema
Prognosis good
Elimination no problem at this time

Activity ambulatory as tolerated
Rehabilitation Potential good
Emotional Status: alert, pleasant, forgetful at times
has three children who live out of state (son, Brian 1-386-407-3810)
Family History & Involvement lives with wife (Jane) in one story home,

PHYSICIAN Dr. A.J. Hayes, Community Med Clinic No. 3-601-845
                                           MR 825-68-8498

PHYSICAL ENVIRONMENT:
  Safety adequate - bed rails Housing bathroom and bedroom on one level
  Sanitation adequate   Transportation car
  Safety Measures no vulnerabilities noted
Patient and Family Teaching yes   Understanding appears adequate
Both patient and wife appear to have understanding of
disease process and are aware of its limitations
Type of Service HHA 12 hours daily and prn
Frequency of Visits RN (Director of Nursing) twice weekly
Required Medical Equipment/Supplies:
  Type stethoscope and blood pressure equipment, hospital bed & rails
  Purpose monitor pts condition, safety, comfort
Need for other Community Resources County Social Services Department
  Action Taken Social worker, public health nurse, Shamrock Director
of Nursing, patient and family will meet to evaluate family
for alternate care grant

DISCHARGE SUMMARY:
  Patient's Condition _____
  Goals Attained _____
  Reason for Termination of Service _____

  Date of Discharge _____
                                              Director of Nursing
                        (over)

Figure 10–8 Sample home care records (Courtesy of Shamrock In-Home Nursing Care, Rochester, MN)

DRUG PROFILE				
Medication	Dosage	Time	Common Side Effects	
Lasix	20 mg	daily	9 AM	
Lanoxin	0.125 mg	daily	9 AM Call office before giving if pulse rate is below 60	
K-lyte	25 meq	daily	9 AM	
Multivitamin	1	daily	9 AM	
Calcec	100 mg	daily	9 AM	

PROBLEM	TREATMENT	GOAL
Potential alternations in respiratory function related to CHF	1. Monitor respiratory rate, effort and quality. 2. Lung sounds per auscultation 1-3 times per day as condition indicates. 3. Check neck veins for distention. 4. Allow pt. to assume position of comfort: fowlers or semi-fowlers position at times of distress. 5. Instruct pt. to take deep breaths and cough 6-8 times per day. 6. Encourage quiet rest periods in the morning and afternoon. 7. Arrange essential supplies within reach of pt. to avoid energy expenditure.	Pt. will adequately demonstrate methods of effective coughing, breathing and energy conservation.

Figure 10–8 (Continued)

PROBLEM	TREATMENT	GOAL

Fluid volume excess: edema related to CHF	8. Eat frequent, small meals to avoid stomach distention and pressure on diaphragm
	 1. Assess pt. knowledge of 90 mEq Na diet
	 2. Instruct pt. on diet and assess compliance
	   a) record daily intake of food and fluid until pt. knowledge and compliance are established
	 3. Daily assessment for dependent venous pooling:
	   a) measure thighs and calves
	   b) check ankles and feet for pitting edema
	   c) check sacral area, face and abdomen for puffiness
	 4. Daily weight (call if greater than 2 lbs/daily)
	 5. Daily intake and output
	 6. Vital signs daily
	 7. Elevate feet when sitting
	 8. Avoid long periods of standing
	 9. Avoid restrictive clothing
	 10. Discourage leg and ankle crossing
	 11. Antiembolism stockings per doctor's order
	   a) apply while lying down
	   b) remove q10 for one hour
		Pt. will have good understanding of factors causing edema and methods to prevent edema. Pt. will exhibit decreased edema.

Figure 10–8 (Continued)

months in a row. But it is not good nursing, or good for you, to become too attached to your patients.

Home health care can be very rewarding. Only you can know what setting will provide the most personal and professional satisfaction.

KEY CONCEPT: RESPONSIBILITIES OF HOME HEALTH CARE NURSES

- Assess safety of home environment.
- Administer treatments and medications as ordered.
- Reinforce patient and family teaching.
- Support family caregiver.
- Document visits and report as directed.
- Function autonomously.

WORKING IN DAY CARE FOR THE ELDERLY OR HANDICAPPED

Responsibilities in a day care setting for the elderly or handicapped individual will be similar to those of a long term care facility. The nurse is responsible for recordkeeping and for giving medications, and sometimes will supervise nursing assistants or volunteers. Family members should be kept informed of any changes noted in the behavior or health status of the day care patient.

Ideally, the people who come to a day care center will come often enough so that you can learn about their individual needs. It has been found that if the center is located in a nursing home, the people attending the center prefer to have their own entrance and own area of the building. Because these people are not ill, only one or two nurses would be needed each day in this setting.

Nursing care of "well" persons still requires attention to their basic needs and to data collection. You may be the one person to notice a subtle change; mentioning it to the person or their family caregiver may prevent a more serious situation from developing. The people in this kind of day care usually are there for the social stimulation as well as basic needs. Your communication skills will get lots of practice!

WORKING IN RESPITE CARE

In Unit 4, respite care was explained. It is practiced in some hospitals. If you are employed in a hospital that has some respite beds, you may be taking care of those patients. Their nursing care will not be different from that given to other patients, with a few exceptions. They are not ill, so the focus of your nursing care should be to keep them as independent as possible. In addition, they have probably brought their own medications with them, but you will be responsible for giving them as ordered. Finally, they are probably paying for this from their own pocket; be economical with supplies.

Mr. Young had a CVA that left him a right-sided hemiplegic. Mrs. Young manages his care at home with occasional assistance from an adult son. When Mrs. Young required a cholecystectomy, she arranged respite care for her husband. This arrangement allowed them to see each other regularly. She could focus her energy on her own recovery without worrying about his care.

Respite care can also be applied to home care situations. Perhaps the family is vacationing and needs someone to stay with a handicapped member. This kind of home respite care may or may not require a nurse. The points discussed earlier about home health care also will apply.

WORKING IN A HOSPICE

The primary responsibility for the bedside nurse in a hospice is to keep the patient comfortable. Implementing the hospice care plan requires close attention to all of the patient's basic needs for physical comfort. Careful positioning, regular turning, and maintaining bowel and bladder functions are all important as comfort measures. Family caregivers are often taught to perform these tasks.

Many hospice patients receive large doses of analgesia by suppository or by IV drip. The analgesia dosage is adjusted according to their comfort level. Hospice patients often remain very alert even with large doses of narcotic analgesics.

Hospices also are concerned about psychological comfort. Whether he is a hospice in-patient or at home, the nurse needs to assess how he and the family are coping with their situation. The emotional stages of the dying experience are very stressful for everyone involved. Your observations will provide important data for the hospice team to use.

Another important part of working with hospice patients is the need for attending workshops, classes, and seminars about pain management and death and dying. It seems that the best hospice nurses are those who have reached their own understanding of the dying process.

KEY CONCEPT: RESPONSIBILITIES OF THE NURSE IN OTHER EXPANDED SETTINGS

- Day care: observe, give delegated treatments and medications, document, pay attention.
- Respite care: maintain the patient's independence, give delegated treatments and medications, be economical.
- Hospice: keep the patient comfortable, both physically and psychologically.

SUMMARY

In most expanded care settings, nurses will continue to use their observation skills. Whether working independently or with a team, nurses are responsible for applying the nursing process to meet the patients' needs. In office settings, communication focuses on data collection. In an ambulatory surgery setting, patient education is vital. Careful assessments are needed in home health care settings.

Nurses also must keep accurate records in any care setting. Documentation is essential for continuity of care as well as for reimbursement. Understanding human behaviors—patients, families, co-workers—remains a vital aspect of nursing.

FOR DISCUSSION

- Interview an office or clinic nurse in your community. What specific skills are needed? Can you obtain those skills?
- Arrange to accompany a home health care nurse on a home visit. What kinds of assessments can you make about the home, the patient, the visit?
- Explore your community for other expanded settings for health care delivery.

Situations for Study

Using the nursing process and the samples in the unit as guides, prepare nursing care plans for the patients in the following settings.

1. You are the clinic nurse
   A. Maria Gonzales is a 23-year-old laboratory technician who is four months pregnant with her second baby. She is engaged to the baby's father, who also fathered her four-year-old son. As you greet her, you notice that she looks very tired. It is 3:30 P.M.

   She began this pregnancy at 112 pounds, and now weighs 120 pounds. Her blood pressure is 102/66, hemoglobin is 12, urinalysis is negative, fetal heart rate is strong and regular at 154.

   What data do you have? What questions would you ask Maria before the doctor comes in?
   B. A week has passed. Maria telephones the clinic at 8:30 A.M. to report that she has been vomiting all night and has abdominal cramps.

   What are some questions you would ask? What would you advise?
2. You are employed in an Ambulatory Surgery Unit

   Gwendolyn Schuster is scheduled for right cataract extraction with implant. She is 78 years old. Information from the doctor states that she is a controlled hypertensive and has osteoarthritis in both knees. Her son brings her to the unit where you are working.

   What kind of a care plan can you develop? Are there specific questions you will ask?
3. You are a Home Health Care Nurse

   Charlie Schmitz is 72 years old. He was hospitalized for a week with an infected ulcer on the bottom of his right foot. He has been a diabetic for 20 years, and has diabetic neuropathy of both feet. His wife is 70 and has mild congestive heart failure. They live in a duplex; their four adult children all live in other parts of the country.

   Mr. Schmitz was found to have adequate circulation to his foot, so the doctor referred him to your agency for home health care until the foot ulcer is healed. The ulcer requires daily soaking in a Betadine solution and repacking with saline dressings. The case coordinator has assigned you to perform this care. Other items in the care plan include reinforcing all aspects of diabetic management. Mr. Schmitz weighs 225 pounds. He is 5 feet 10 inches tall. He takes an oral hypoglycemic tablet daily.

You arrive for your initial visit at 10 A.M. The Schmitzes have just finished breakfast, which you observe consisted of bacon, pancakes with syrup, grapefruit halves, and coffee. They offer you coffee.

What data is useful? How will you proceed?

4. You are the nurse in an Adult Day Care Center

   George Little is a 68-year-old widower. He lives with a married son. He had a cerebrovascular accident three years ago that left him with residual paralysis of his right arm. He also is dysphasic, but can communicate fairly well in simple words if you don't rush him. He walks with a cane. Mr. Little's daughter-in-law brings him to the Day Care Center at 8:30 A.M. four days each week. His son comes for him at 4:30 P.M.

What are priority needs for Mr. Little while he is at the Center? What areas will need special nursing attention?

5. You are a Home Health Care Nurse

   You are assigned to visit a new family in town who has been referred by a school nurse. Use the theory of basic needs as a guide in developing a care plan. This is the data you have collected:

   > There was an old woman
   >   who lived in a shoe.
   > She had so many children
   >   she didn't know what to do.
   > She gave them some broth,
   >   without any bread,
   > whipped them all soundly
   >   and put them to bed.

11

Nurse's Responsibilities to Self and Career

OBJECTIVES:

After completing this unit, you will be able to:

- Discuss the importance of assessing personal needs related to employment.
- Define resumé and explain its purpose.
- List steps in preparing for an interview.
- Explain the purpose of liability insurance.
- Discuss the importance of continuing education.
- Identify three issues nurses must face.

The previous unit discussed some of the responsibilities nurses will have in expanded health care delivery settings. This unit will review how important it is to understand yourself when you seek that first position, figure 11–1. Finding the job that fits you is vital to personal satisfaction. The importance of continuing your education after you are licensed will be covered. Finally, some issues in nursing and in society will be considered.

UNDERSTANDING YOURSELF

Nursing education includes some basic psychology and the discussion of human behaviors. You have even applied some of those concepts to patient care. It is also important to apply them to yourself.

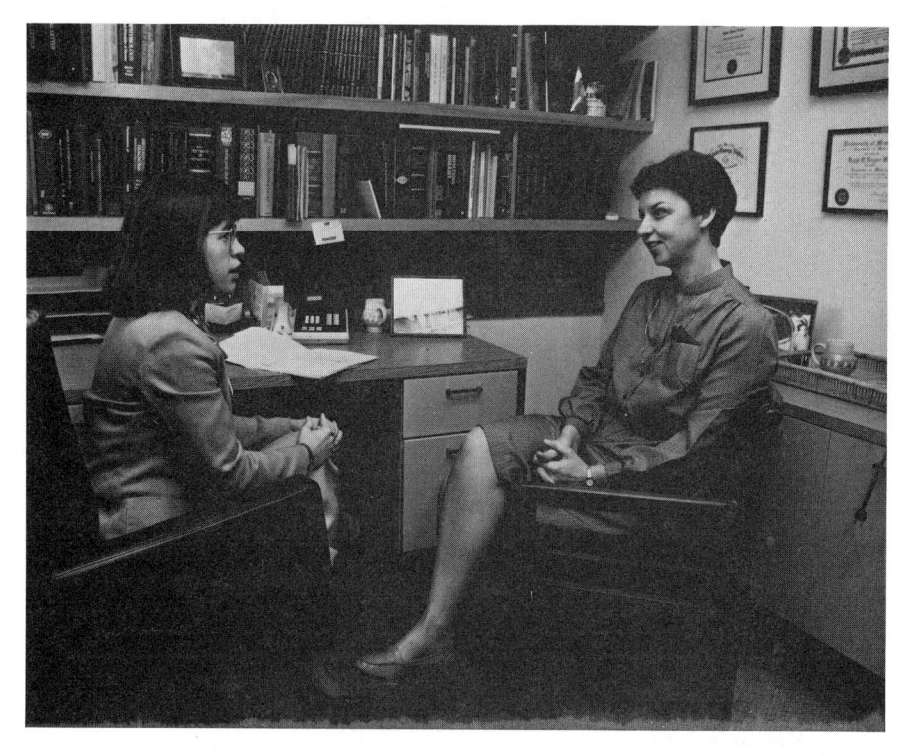

Figure 11–1 Physician interviews nurse applicant

What makes you tick? Do you really enjoy working with people? Would you prefer working with machines? What are your strengths? Weaknesses? How will your work fit with the rest of your life? Do you have family responsibilities that will limit your choices of work hours or locations?

When you have thought about yourself in this way, you will be able to realistically look at the various settings that employ nurses and see which is most appealing to you. Consider what setting will offer the most personal satisfaction and opportunity for growth. You may enjoy the busy activity of a hospital. A classmate may prefer the one-on-one relationships developed in home health care. Another classmate may be a "born leader" and be happiest in a supervisory setting.

As you mature as a person and as a nurse, your needs may change. It is very common for changes to occur. The world will continue to change, too; in five or ten years there may be nursing positions that are not available today. Seeking new employment can be an adventure, and a growth experience.

Perhaps you will stay with one position for several years and not realize that it no longer provides satisfaction. You should be aware of potential burnout and recognize the symptoms, figure 11–2. *Burnout* has come to mean exhaustion. People who work full time in highly stressful settings are particularly vulnerable. You may just need to take some extra time off. Sometimes people find they need to change their type of work entirely. In order to be the most effective nurse for your patients, you must first consider your own needs and see that they are met.

It is well known that many nurses, especially those with young children, may choose not to be employed. This may be a temporary or permanent situation. Some nursing graduates find they are happier in another kind of employment. No matter where your future path lies, your nursing education is valuable and will influence you and your family for the rest of your life.

KEY CONCEPT: KNOW THYSELF!

- Consider your own strengths and weaknesses.
- Consider your other responsibilities.
- Analyze what you need for job satisfaction.
- Recognize the potential for personal growth and change.
- Avoid burnout.

Unusual fatigue

Irritability

Insomnia

Preoccupation with your work

Weight loss or gain

Picking fights with loved ones

Vague physical complaints

Figure 11–2 Burnout warning!

JOB SEEKING

Resumés

Looking for a job can be an exciting time if you are well prepared. The steps to follow are listed in figure 11-3. One thing you should do before applying for that first position is to prepare a resumé. A *resumé* is a one or two-page document that describes you, your skills and interests. Potential employers are usually impressed with a neat resumé, so take the time to do it right. Your school may assist you with this, or you may seek help from a specialist in the field. Sample resumés are included as figures 11-4 and 11-5.

When you are completing an employment application, be as concise and as neat as possible. Answer each item truthfully. You may wish to include a copy of nursing competencies with the application if your program supplies you with that information. Sometimes new graduates are frustrated when every advertised position says, "Experience necessary." Employers always want experienced workers, but they don't always find them. If you really want the position, pursue it vigorously!

Interviews

The next step is usually an interview. Prepare for the interview by learning all you can about the institution or agency. Think ahead about the questions

---

1. Read employment ads. Talk to other nurses about possible jobs. Decide what kind of job you want.
2. Send a letter of inquiry in response to advertised opening, or to see if an opening exists. Include resumé.
3. Make a telephone call to arrange appointment for interview. (10 days after letter, or in response to the employer's letter.)
4. Complete the employment application.
5. Interview. Arrive 10 minutes early. Be calm. Have some questions prepared.
6. Send a thank you letter. Accept the offer, decline the offer, ask when they will decide about the position. The acceptance letter should verify the date and time that employment is to begin.

Figure 11-3 Steps in job-seeking

JOHN JONES
1500 Elm Street
Yourtown, MN 55XXX
(XXX) 555-XXXX

CAREER OBJECTIVE:	Practical Nurse position with opportunity to use technical and communication skills
EDUCATION:	Community Vocational Technical Institute Yourtown, MN 55XXX Practical Nursing Program (11 months) Graduate June 1986 * Director's List for academic achievement * Grade Point Average 3.5

Significant Courses:

Anatomy and Physiology	Maternal Health
Nursing I and II	Child Health
Pharmacology	Medical–Surgical Nursing
First Aid	
CPR	Gerontology
Clinical Experience 550 hours	Community and Home Health

Yourtown High School, Yourtown, MN 55XXX
Graduated May 1985
B Honor Roll during 3 high school years

Significant Courses:

Biology	Health Occupations
Psychology	Computer Science

WORK EXPERIENCE: Family owned corner grocery. I shared tasks with parents, two brothers, one sister, and learned all aspects of a small business. I developed communication skills while working with customers.

ACTIVITIES:
Volunteer:
    Assistant Explorer Scout Leader
    Red Cross Bloodmobile
Community Hockey Team

Hobbies: running, fishing, photography

Figure 11–4 Example of a resumé for a PN/VN position

REFERENCES: Lucille Brown, Director
              Practical Nursing Program
              Community Vocational Technical Institute
              Yourtown, MN 55XXX (XXX) 555-XXXX

              Mary Chase, Health Occupations Teacher
              Yourtown High School
              Yourtown, MN 55XXX (XXX) 555-XXXX

Figure 11–4 (Continued)

JANE DOE
1940 Oak Drive
Anytown, MN 55XXX
(XXX) 555-XXXX

CAREER OBJECTIVE: Primary nurse position using technical, communication, and nursing skills with goal of future management.

EDUCATION: Community Vocational Technical Institute
             Yourtown, MN 55XXXX
             Practical Nursing Program (11 months)
             Graduate June 1986
             * Director's List for academic achievement
             * Grade Point Average 3.8

Significant Courses

Anatomy and Physiology	Maternal Health
Nursing I and II	Child Health
Pharmacology	Medical–Surgical Nursing
First Aid	
CPR	Gerontology
Clinical Experience 550 hours	Community and Home Health

Community College, Ourtown, MN 1973–1975
Associate of Arts Degree in Accounting
Grade Point Average of 3.5

Figure 11–5 Example of a resumé for a PN/VN position

WORK EXPERIENCE:	Anytown Physicians Clinic	1980–1984
	Anytown, MN 55XXX	
	Clinic Office Staff—responsible for computerized billing, insurance forms, and liasion with patients for billing information	
	Johnson Department Store	1976–1979
	Ourtown, MN 55XXX	
	Junior Accountant—responsible for payroll and billing with a small firm	
VOLUNTEER WORK:	Red Cross volunteer, coordinating community Bloodmobile	
	Girl Scouts, assist with special projects	
PERSONAL:	Active member of Anytown Community Theater	
	Avid jogger and needlepoint enthusiast	
REFERENCES:	Available on request.	

Figure 11–5 (Continued)

you might ask: How much orientation is given before you are on your own? What is their average daily census? What is the usual staffing ratio? What opportunities are there for advancement? Perhaps you have special needs, such as requesting future time off for your honeymoon.

It is believed that employers often decide on a potential employee within the first few minutes of the interview. This means you must pay attention to your appearance. Wearing blue jeans is NOT acceptable, even when you are only requesting an application form.

Be sure to be on time for the interview. Be aware of the influence of body language; be alert, stand and sit using good posture. Don't chew gum or smoke. Be confident. You know you're a good nurse.

Employment policies should be explained to you at the interview. You can ask for a copy of the job description. Examples are given in figures 11–6 and 11–7. Be prepared to point out your strengths.

You have a right to expect honesty from the potential employer. It is important for yourself and for nursing that you seek employment with a reputable agency. You are a nurse, and your work represents nursing. When you accept a job, you become a representative of that employer.

POSITION: <u>LICENSED PRACTICAL NURSE</u>

PURPOSE: To give comprehensive patient care as assigned by Director of Nursing.

Qualifications: Currently licensed as L.P.N. in State of Minnesota.

Current license number and expiration date on file in office. Two years experience in the nursing field.

Accountable To: Patient and Family
SHAMROCK DIRECTOR OF NURSING

<u>PRINCIPAL DUTIES:</u>

Provides comprehensive care in accord with established policies and procedures of Shamrock In-Home Nursing Care and consults with Director of Nursing regarding any changes in care plan.

Care Includes:

Administration of medications and treatments as ordered by the physician EXCEPT:

- *No* anti coagulants by injection
- *No* I.V. push medication
- *No* insulin
- *No* calculated doses by injection

Physical and psychological care.

Patient and family education.

Recognizes and interprets symptoms and institutes remedial measures within the legal limits of Licensed Practical Nursing in the State of Minnesota and reports significant changes in patient's condition to the Director of Nursing immediately.

Records observations completely, accurately, legibly, and concisely.

Figure 11–6 Sample home health job description for LP/VN (Courtesy of Shamrock In-Home Nursing Care, Rochester, MN)

> Maintain record of patient's condition, nursing care, patient's response to care, patient and family education in:
>
> > Nurses' notes
> > All other required forms
>
> Maintain the patient's room and equipment necessary for his/her care and safety.
>
> Adapts to the family standards and their home environment.
>
> Demonstrates and teaches sound home health practices and management.
>
> Assist patient in arrangements for medical appointments, shopping, errands, money management, etc.
>
> Participates in inservice and utilizes outside resources for own continuing professional education.
>
> Participates in regular performance evaluation of self with Directors of Nursing.
>
> Ability to work with team concept of nursing.
>
> Ability to accept and utilize supervision.

Figure 11-6 (Continued)

The First Job

It may be necessary to accept a first position that is not your first choice. Consider it as a learning experience and be patient. Allow yourself several months in any position before even trying to decide whether or not it is right for you. Then, if you decide you would like to try something else, wait a few more months. Try to stay with the first job for one year. Employers frown on resumés that show a history of frequent job changes. When you do decide to change jobs, follow the proper resignation policy. Most employers appreciate both the verbal statement and a letter of resignation with at least two weeks advance notice. You may be asked to stay until a replacement can be hired and oriented. NEVER walk off a job.

During this time of job-seeking activity, review your notes or book references about the basic rules of nursing ethics which you have been taught. You also should obtain a copy of your state's Nurse Practice Act

POSITION: REGISTERED NURSE

Purpose: To give comprehensive patient care as assigned by the Director of Nursing.

Qualifications: Currently licensed as an R.N. in the State of Minnesota
    Current license number and expiration date on file in office.

Experience—Two years in nursing field.

Accountable To: Patient and Family
SHAMROCK DIRECTOR OF NURSING

PRINCIPAL DUTIES:

Plans, provides and evaluates nursing care in accord with established policies and procedures of Shamrock; and consults with the Directors of Nursing regarding any changes in care plan.

Care Includes:
  Administration of medications and treatments as ordered by the physician
  Physical and psychological care
  Patient and family education

Recognizes and interprets symptoms and institutes remedial measures within the legal limits of nursing practice within the State of Minnesota; and report significant changes in patient's condition to the Director of Nursing immediately.

Exercises professional judgment in adapting nursing measures to changing needs.

Maintains accurate and complete records of patient condition, nursing care, patient's response to care, patient/family education in:
  Nurses' notes
  All other required forms

Maintains patient's room and equipment necessary for his care and safety.

Figure 11-7 Sample home health job description for an RN (Courtesy of Shamrock In-Home Nursing Care, Rochester, MN)

> Adapts to family standards and their home environment.
>
> Demonstrates and teaches sound home health practices and management.
>
> Assists patient in arranging medical appointments, shopping, errands, money management, etc.
>
> Participates in scheduled patient conferences with Directors of Nursing.
>
> Contributes to ongoing formulation of nursing care plans.
>
> Participates in inservice and utilizes outside resources for own continuing professional education.
>
> Participates in regular performance evaluation of self with Directors of Nursing.
>
> Ability to work with team concept of nursing.
>
> Ability to accept and utilize supervision.

Figure 11-7 (Continued)

to be aware of your legal limitations. If you are unable to find a copy, contact your State Board or Department of Nursing.

Liability Insurance

Liability insurance for nurses is available through nursing organizations or independent agencies. Liability insurance offers protection from payment of damages charged to you if a patient should sue. The insurance company agrees to handle the case for the nurse.

Investigate how much insurance your employer provides. Then decide if you need additional coverage. Liability insurance provided by the employer will only protect you while you are at work. You may want to invest in an individual policy if you want coverage for the rest of the time. When responsibilities include the supervision of others, you are liable for their actions as well as your own.

Nurse practitioners and specialists are finding liability insurance very expensive. Many nurses carry insurance so that they are protected while they are not working, too. You must make a personal decision about your need for liability insurance. It will depend on the kind of work you do and your own resources.

Labor Unions

In some parts of the country, nurses employed in hospitals and long term care facilities have joined labor unions. Labor unions are organizations of workers. The Union is concerned with salaries, benefits, and other aspects of improving working conditions.

If union membership is required for employment, the job situation is called *closed shop*. If you are not required to join the labor union, you may be charged a percentage of dues as your "fair share" because you benefit from the labor union's employment contract. Nursing organizations may be concerned with employment contracts, but membership also includes other benefits.

Continuing Education

After graduation from a nursing program, you may think you've had enough education for awhile. Everyone continues to learn daily. Some positions will require mastery of additional skills, such as computer keyboarding, drawing blood samples, or taking x-rays. Your employer may offer workshops and meetings designed to keep your skills current. Take advantage of every opportunity to expand your knowledge. In this shrinking world, it may be useful to learn a second (or even a third) language. Other communication skills can also be improved through taking specific courses. You may consider studying management skills. Many of the areas included in your nursing curriculum were introductory courses. You can find enrichment courses through adult education programs, community colleges, universities, and nursing organizations.

In some States, nurses are required to show evidence of a certain number of *Continuing Education Units* (CEUs) for relicensure. If this is true in your state, it will be necessary to attend classes for the required number of hours within the allotted amount of time. In Minnesota, RNs need to obtain 30 CEUs in two years. Some states require CEUs for LP/VNs as well. One CEU is equal to one hour of approved classtime or workshop related to nursing.

So far, we have addressed continuing your education because of the job or licensure requirements. You may wish to pursue more education just for fun. Developing a new hobby, learning Chinese cooking or calligraphy are also ways to continue growing as an individual.

UNIT 11/NURSE'S RESPONSIBILITIES TO SELF AND CAREER

KEY CONCEPT: SEEKING AND KEEPING JOBS

- Resumés are tools to help get an interview.
- Interviews provide a chance to ask questions.
- Try to stay with your first job for at least one year.
- Liability insurance protects on and off the job.
- Labor Unions strive to improve working conditions, including salaries.
- Learning does not stop with graduation.

ISSUES TO CONSIDER

Ethical Conflicts in Nursing

Nurses are expected to follow certain standards, which are nursing ethics. *Ethics*, you will recall, refers to a code of conduct and morals. Points included in nursing ethics are listed in figure 11–8.

Sometimes nurses will find conflict between the ethics they have been taught and the responsibilities they are given. These conflicts often involve relationships with others. Perhaps a patient may refuse a treatment that you know is needed. This creates a conflict between your responsibility to

- Nurses respect their patients and care for them regardless of race, sex, creed, ethnic or socioeconomic background.
- Nurses protect the privacy of their patients.
- Nurses are responsible for their own actions.
- Nurses contribute to efforts to protect the public from misinformation and incompetent practitioners.
- Nurses accept only the payment for their work as contracted.

Figure 11–8 Nurses' ethics

carry out the treatment and your respect for the patient's right to refuse treatment.

Maintaining the patient's right to privacy may create a conflict if the disease could be a public health concern. Sometimes a doctor's order conflicts with the patient's wishes; what can the nurse do then? Or a nurse becomes aware that a colleague is incompetent. Should loyalty to your co-worker take priority if there is a risk to patients?

You can apply a basic problem-solving procedure when faced with an ethical conflict:

(1) Collect as much data as possible. Try to be objective. Check policy handbooks and state laws, if needed.
(2) Define the issue creating the conflict. Be as specific as possible.
(3) Seek appropriate advice. This may mean talking with a supervisor, a peer, a lawyer, or member of the clergy.
(4) Consider possible actions and their consequences. This may take some time.
(5) Take action. You must be prepared to accept the results of the action taken.

Figure 11–9 summarizes this problem-solving method.

The Women's Movement

Nursing began as an extension of the woman's traditional roles of caring and nurturing in the family. Even though there were men in nursing from the beginning (priests, monks, soldiers), and there are men in nursing today, it remains predominantly female work.

---

1. Collect data.
2. Identify the issue.
3. Seek advice from others.
4. Consider all possible actions, including the consequences of each.
5. Take action.

Figure 11–9 The steps of a problem-solving method

Nursing advances in the United States paralleled the advances that women were making in society. Some people state that many of the problems nurses have had with assertiveness, autonomy, low pay, and even recognition as a separate health profession stem from the fact that most nurses are women.

It is true that nursing needs more men. As society opens its "male" occupations to women, "female" occupations should also be made available to men. Male and female nurses bring different perspectives to nursing, resulting in growth and change for all nurses.

The nurse who respects and accepts patients should also be able to respect and accept other nurses, whatever their race or gender. This is a goal worthy of us all.

Bio-ethical Issues

Bio-ethical issues are those situations that create problems for society because of new medical technology. Machinery has affected life. Technology has advanced faster than human laws can handle it. The ethics of using available machinery to affect life presents problems at times.

Nurses who work closely with patients are often asked for their opinions. You will not be in a position to make ethical decisions for a patient, but you do need to understand the kinds of questions that can arise. It is not ethical to tell the patient or family what to do. It is important that you listen to them and help them sort out their feelings in order to make a decision. Be alert to cues that indicate they need to be referred to the doctor or a member of the clergy. Your communication skills are very important.

You are already aware of many bio-ethical dilemmas. Abortion, euthanasia, organ transplantation—the list could go on and on. People's values and religious beliefs make decisions very difficult. You need to consider these areas of controversy from your own value system, too. But whatever your personal opinion is, you must accept the patient's decision.

Perhaps you are a home health nurse assigned to care for an elderly widower. Your specific care involves monitoring his blood pressure, making sure he takes his medications, and reinforcing diabetic instructions. One day he tells you that his son has read about diabetics who need dialysis treatments. He asks you what that means, and whether he will ever need it. How can you answer?

Technical versus Professional Nursing

One of the issues facing nurses during the rest of this century is the controversy about kinds of nurses. There is no national consensus at this time about what educational requirements will be needed for what role.

You are being educated as a bedside nurse. Your knowledge and skills will always be valued. Your license cannot be revoked because of changing educational standards.

Technicians in any field practice between the major decision makers with in-depth knowledge, and the employees who learn on the job. Some nurses resent the technician label, but others accept it willingly.

There will be some changes in nursing education by the turn of the century. You need to be aware of that. More education will be required for all health care workers. One change may well involve the titles and requirements of nurses. Whether those changes will affect your role will depend on legislation in your particular state. It may be to your advantage to continue your education in a structured way, seeking an additional degree or credential if that is what you want.

KEY CONCEPT: ISSUES REQUIRE ATTENTION

- Potential conflict of nursing ethics may occur.
- The women's movement has affected nursing.
- Bio-ethical dilemmas grow out of use of technology.
- Technical vs. professional nursing: what changes will take place?

SUMMARY

Understanding your own strengths and weaknesses is as important to your job satisfaction as the job itself. Study your strengths and abilities, then investigate potential positions before you apply. Realize that your first position is only a start, not where you'll be in the future.

Graduating as a nurse is a big accomplishment. But, it is only the beginning of your education. Keeping your skills current is vital to your practice. Further education may be desirable for your work, your license, or for fun. Nurses need to know about many concerns that affect them, including ethical problems, the women's movement, and the future of nursing.

FOR DISCUSSION

- Write a paragraph discussing the kind of nursing position you would like to have, including reasons. Share your ideas with your classmates.
- What kinds of continuing education for nurses is available in your community? Will you be required to have CEUs for relicensure?
- Talk to an insurance agent about liability insurance for nurses. What is available? What does it cover? What does it cost?
- Are nurses unionized in your area? What do you know about labor unions?
- Suppose you see another nurse hit a patient. What should you do?
- A doctor tells you to not attempt resuscitation of a patient, but refuses to write the order. What are your options and responsibilities?

QUESTIONS FOR REVIEW

1. Give three reasons for studying your own needs before you start seeking a job.
2. What is a resumé? What is it for?
3. List the steps in preparing for a job interview.
4. What is the purpose of liability insurance?
5. List three issues facing nurses.

12

Nurses' Influencing Future Health Care

OBJECTIVES:

After completing this unit, you will be able to:

- Discuss formal and informal ways nurses promote health.
- Discuss quality health care issues and philosophies.
- Identify four ways nurses can contribute to quality health care.
- Explain ways that nurses can become more aware of health care issues.
- Identify five organizations that are concerned with health care issues.

This unit will discuss the importance of every nurse's awareness of health care issues in order to make an impact on future health care in this country. One of the major issues of the '80s and '90s will be that of quality care. How can nurses contribute to that discussion? How can nurses make sure that every patient receives quality care?

The second issue, which is closely related to quality care, is that of access. Access to care includes the geographical distribution of health care. It also includes the issue of costs, which threatens to make health care unaffordable for many people. What can nurses do to make a difference?

Ways that nurses promote health will be discussed. Organizations for nurses and for health concerns will be reviewed. Political involvement of nurses, both within nursing and within the greater community, will also be considered.

HEALTH PROMOTION

Health promotion, you will recall from Unit 2, is the first level of intervention. Some examples of health promotion include government regulations that monitor the quality of our food, air, water, and environment. Another example is health education which is aimed at the entire population. Some of this education is presented through the media, such as campaigns to encourage drivers to use seat belts. Other education is done through schools, as when pre-schoolers are taught to wash their hands before eating.

Nurses' Formal Roles

Nurses are often employed by businesses as wellness consultants or occupational health nurses. These positions usually require a baccalaureate degree. Such nurses include general health education as part of that type of job. Teaching about safety practices on the job and healthy lifestyles could fall into the nurse's role.

Newspapers, magazines, and radio and television stations often employ a doctor or nurse, either full time or part time as a consultant. A nurse in that position could have a great impact on the health education of the audience. For example, when the President of the United States has a health problem, the media present all the ramifications of it in minute detail. The "health reporter" has a responsibility to explain the problem in terms that the public can understand. Explanations that will inform people without creating alarm are very helpful.

Nurses who become practitioners and have their own practice are also working in Level I much of the time. The education they give their patients will often fall into health promotion. A young woman may visit a midwife for information about birth control. She will also benefit from a general discussion about healthy diet and lifestyle practices. Later in her life, she will have a healthier pregnancy and baby if she learns how to take care of herself now.

Governmental units that make regulations about the environment often use health workers as consultants. When new regulations are proposed, there are public hearings. The nurse who works as a health consultant is usually a public health nurse (PHN).

Nurses' Informal Roles

For the new graduate the role in health promotion will probably fall into the informal category. Your education and license to practice nursing makes your knowledge very valuable. Most people automatically respect the knowledge and expertise of nurses, so you will always serve as a health consultant, even when you're not aware of it!

Everyone you meet in your role as a nurse may be influenced by what you say and do. Wherever you work, patients and their families will look to you to explain things that the doctor or another health professional has said. You may have already found yourself giving those explanations. Someone taking Lithium Carbonate for treatment of manic-depression may admit to skipping a few doses because they feel well. Your comment about the importance of continuing medication to "even out those ups and downs" will be heard, and the patient benefits from the explanation.

The people in the rest of your life will be influenced by you, too. Sometimes it is hard to be a role model for a healthy lifestyle, but that's still part of the role. That doesn't mean you have to walk around wearing a halo! It just means that you should be aware of your influence. That's why nurses who smoke cigarettes don't do it at the nurses' station.

Some nurses may have *inactive licensure,* that is, not be employed as nurses. Other nurses may maintain their licensure but be temporarily unemployed, or may choose not to be employed as a nurse. All of these nurses still maintain their influence regarding health concerns among their families and friends. Certainly, parenting presents many opportunities to teach children healthy lifestyles and attitudes.

It may sometimes be surprising to hear the kinds of questions people ask nurses. "Will I really lose a tooth with every baby I have?" "My sister has three boys, and I'm stuck with four girls. I just don't understand." "Only fat people have high blood pressure." "Isn't everyone over 70 senile?"

Another aspect of your informal role is your responsibility to be aware of events that relate to health issues in your community. If the local landfill is seeking permission to expand, you should try to learn more about it and attend the public hearing. How close to homes will the new area be? What kind of drainage exists? Are there private wells nearby? At such a hearing, you cannot speak for the health system, but your knowledge of health problems makes your input valued as that of an informed citizen, figure 12–1.

Because of the changes in the health care delivery system, Americans will be facing many more choices about their health care. Nurses can be invaluable resources in helping people make these choices. Not everyone knows about nurse practitioners, for example, and the kinds of health care that they can provide. Consumers also may need guidance in seeking home health care or finding the right kind of help for their family situation. You can use your knowledge of the available services in your community to help them.

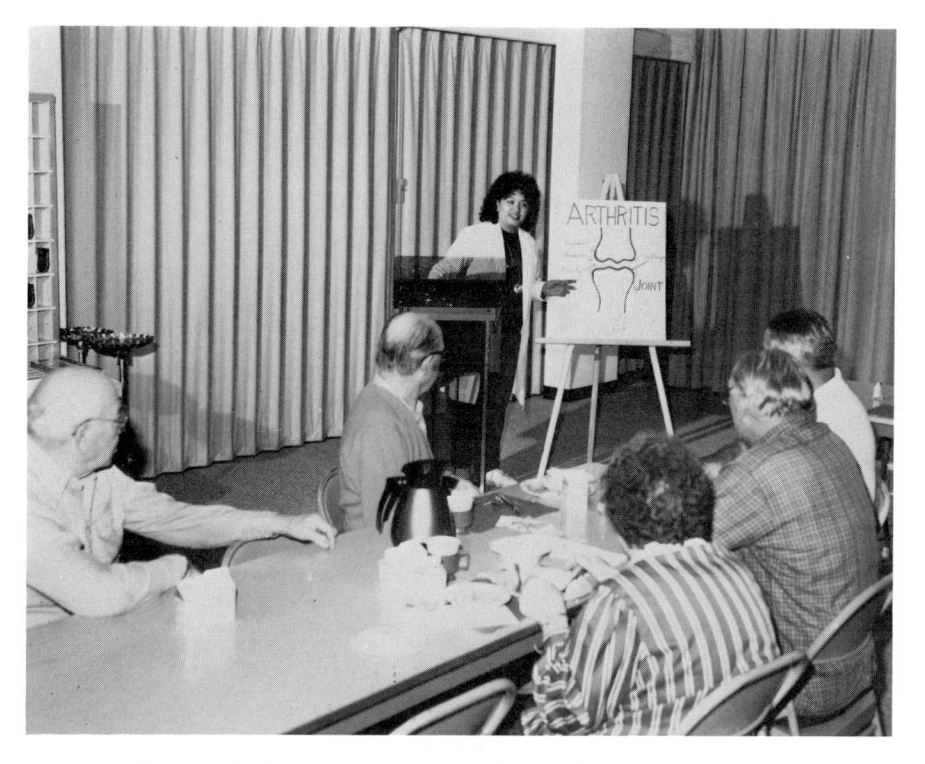

Figure 12–1 The nurse as a community resource person

KEY CONCEPT: YOU WILL ASSIST IN HEALTH PROMOTION

- Formally—employment as health consultants in business, industry, and government; nurse practitioners
- Informally—explanations to patients, families, friends and acquaintances; role models of lifestyles; solutions to local health issues because of education

ISSUES OF QUALITY CARE AND ACCESS

Many people have identified quality of health care as a key issue that needs to be addressed. One might wonder why quality is an issue, if the nation really has an excess of physicians. If there are so many empty hospital beds, the remaining patients should have really good care. Yet the quality question remains.

The issue of access to health care is closely related to a discussion of quality care. Access means availability. This includes the distribution of health care providers and personnel. It also includes concerns about the costs of health care. Third party payers are raising their monthly fees for the insured. Some also have deductible clauses, where the insured must pay the first $50–$500 claimed each year. This is true for private insurance plans as well as government programs.

What is quality health care? Who should make decisions? Who is eligible to have it? What can nurses do about it?

Economic Philosophy

There are some who view health care as an industry, a business in which profit is the bottom line. Economists say that any services that do not show profit must be cut. Each new service offered will compete with other services; the one the consumers prefer will succeed. These business people measure quality of care as the number of people served for the cost. A quality hospital will serve many people and make money.

This philosophy governs the rest of the marketplace, and the health care industry is just beginning to learn how it works. Sometimes there are segments of the market that cannot show a profit, however, and those areas will be lost. This philosophy may work for selling soft drinks or cars, but whether it can be adapted to health care services remains uncertain.

What will happen to the millions of Americans who only have limited geographical access to health care? What will happen to people who cannot afford the deductible portion of their insurance? What will happen to the people who do not have medical insurance? Will the changes in society cause these numbers to grow?

Nurses need to understand the economic pressures faced by their patients. Unit 3 discussed methods of paying for health care; you should be aware of your patient's payment arrangements. Helping the patient and family learn how to manage dressing changes, for example, can eliminate some of the visits made by the home health nurse. That will save the patient money.

Nurses need to understand the economic pressures faced by their employers, too. Vendors must be paid, the heat and light bills must be paid, and salaries must be paid. Careful use of supplies will help your employer control costs. Thorough documentation of treatments will help insure reimbursement from a third party payer.

Quality at Any Cost

Comprehensive health care is viewed by some persons as the right of every American. They consider medicine and nursing as social goods. This philosophy attempts to meet everyone's health needs. Advocates of a National Health Policy claim that health services should be standardized across the country so that no one is left out. Quality care, in this view, means that all citizens will have access to whatever health service they need. Services will be evenly distributed and those costs not met by insurance will be borne by taxes.

In order to implement this kind of care, further changes would be needed in the delivery system. Perhaps many more clinics would have to be established in presently under-served areas. The government would have to subsidize much more of the care. Perhaps there would be special hospitals and other services provided only for people who do not have health care insurance. There might also be hospitals specializing in only certain conditions.

Costs of health care are not a major concern for those who have this viewpoint. Research about ways to improve health is very expensive, but very important. The first recipients of artificial hearts could not live outside of the hospital, and all died within two years. However, researchers learned from each one. They will continue to work; eventually someone will receive an artificial heart and live a relatively normal life for many years.

Balancing Cost Containment and Quality Care

Cost containment advocates claim that quality care is not compromised by their efforts. Yet rumors of declining quality abound. Sometimes a patient may be discharged from a hospital and need to be readmitted due to complications. Is this evidence of inadequate care?

Quality of health care from this perspective means that a person will have the best care possible within the constraints of sensible economics. If this involves making choices about life and death, the patient and family must be included in the decision-making process. These choices might include whether to perform surgery for repair of a heart valve if the patient is physically and mentally handicapped. Opponents of this approach claim that it will limit health care to those who can afford it, or that services will be rationed.

Another aspect of this approach is to eliminate the duplication of services now available, especially in large urban areas. Hospitals in many parts of the country have already examined their services and begun combining resources to improve efficiency. It may be wiser for one hospital to have an obstetric unit, instead of six hospitals competing for business. Maybe the home health care units could operate with less confusion and expense if they were merged. Table 12–1 gives an example of this concept.

The idea of large urban hospitals coordinating their services is good for the people who live there. But what will happen in rural America, where communities of 2000 to 5000 people want to have their own hospital? Cost analysts claim that many small community hospitals should close. Many have closed. Some communities no longer have a physician. Some community hospitals have become very progressive, adding services such as Adult Day Care, Respite, and/or Hospice services. These new services may help the hospital be economically successful. Some smaller hospitals will find ways to cooperate with nearby institutions in order to control costs.

The survival of some hospitals in smaller towns will also depend on their distance from larger service areas. Two or three physicians in family practice may serve an area of 6000 people. If they are more than fifty miles from another hospital, the community hospital will probably survive. Consultant specialists might visit the area when needed. Patients with complex problems could be transferred to a larger hospital. In sparsely populated areas, health care may be delivered mostly through a clinic setting. Nurses and a doctor may do much more in home health care. Patients requiring hospitalization would be flown by helicopter to the hospital.

The concerns about costs will not go away in the future. Increasing technology and specialization will make cost-awareness even more important. Yet, these factors should also make services more accessible, and decreases costs. Increasing health care costs, at the present rates, could bankrupt the nation by the year 2050.

It is essential that less expensive ways to deliver care be found. Researchers are developing a simpler way to test for blood cholesterol, for example. The test could be used as a screening tool. The more expensive testing process would then be used only for those who show evidence of high levels.

Nurses' Influence in Quality of Care

Be the best nurse you can be. No matter what the setting, or what patients you care for, be commited to giving quality care. This means understanding and taking care of yourself, too.

Table 12-1 Competitive model vs. cooperative model of hospital services

SOME CITY, USA   Population: 150,000   Hospitals: 6
Practicing Physicians: 115   Practicing Nurses: 950

COMPETITIVE MODEL

Hospital	A	B	C
Beds	1200	150	2000
Specialties	Neuro-Surg	OB	Hospice
Other services	General Med-Surgical Neuro OB Peds Ortho Rehab	Peds Gynecology General Med-Surg Home health	OB Peds General Med-Surg Oncology Urology Home health

Hospital	D	E	F
Beds	550	1500	3500
Specialties	Mental health	Rehab	Coronary surgery
Other services	Neuro Home health	Ortho Neuro	General Med-Surgical Home health OB Peds Hospice

COOPERATIVE MODEL

Hospital	A	B	D
Beds	1100	150	1800
Specialties	Neuro-Surg	OB & Peds	Oncology & Hospice
Other services	General Med-Surgical Neuro Ortho	Home health for Peds & OB	Home health & Hospice

Hospital	D	E	F
Beds	450	1200	3000
Specialties	Mental Health	Rehab	Coronary surgery
Other services	Out-patient mental health clinics	Ortho Neuro	General Med-Surgical Home health

Keep your knowledge and skills current. Continue to learn about the field of nursing where you work, about people, about life. Read nursing and health care magazines and books, ask questions, let people know you're interested in learning. Attend workshops.

Watch for new roles for nurses. Entrepreneurs in nursing may find new ways to promote health and prevent costly hospitalizations. Some nurses are becoming parish nurses, working for churches. Some nurses are becoming block nurses, available for neighborhood health management.

Be aware of social concerns. Pay attention to health care issues in your area. Are there people with unmet health care needs? Be a participant in your community.

Use your influence to help the people around you. People listen to nurses, especially when they know the nurse is a concerned, caring person. Perhaps a therapeutic diet or a medication needs clarification. Sometimes helping means encouraging a neighbor with an annoying symptom to see a doctor. Many times it means just listening.

Figure 12–2 illustrates nurses' influence by intake and output of information.

INTAKE OF INFORMATION

- Informal Education
- Formal Education
- Nursing Organizations
- Community Involvement
- Listening to People
- Reading Journals
- Asking Questions
- Observations
- Awareness

NURSES

OUTPUT OF INFLUENCE

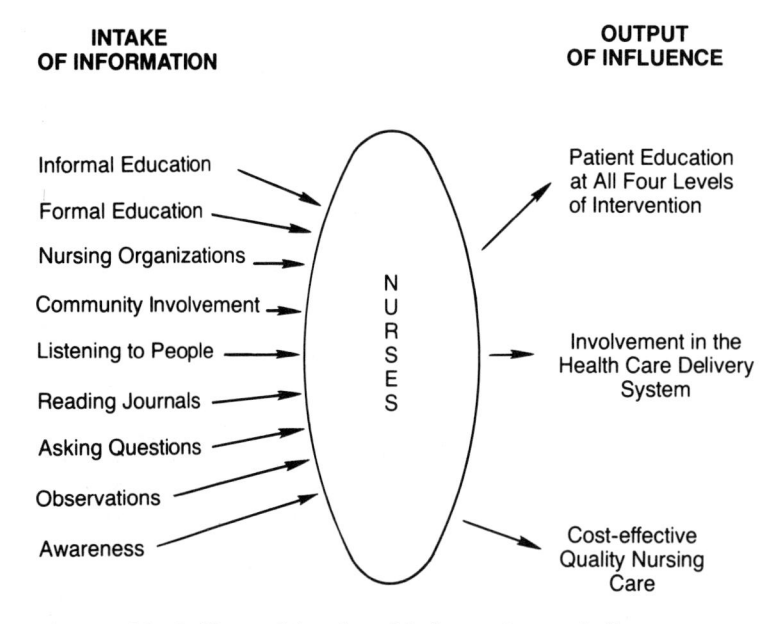

- Patient Education at All Four Levels of Intervention
- Involvement in the Health Care Delivery System
- Cost-effective Quality Nursing Care

Figure 12–2 Nurses' intake of information to influence care

> ### KEY CONCEPT: QUALITY VERSUS COSTS
>
> - Quality may be measured in terms of money spent, number of people served, degree of service received, or some combination of terms.
> - Access includes financial and geographic availability.
> - Cost containment will have to be balanced with quality care.
> - Nurses can contribute to economical quality care by being competent, efficient, and aware of their influence.

POLITICAL INVOLVEMENT

Politics is usually used in reference to government. It also includes the power arrangement of any group: business, professional, family. Politics exist whenever people attempt to work together. Being aware of the political structure of any group is important to your effective action within that group.

Personal Awareness

While learning to be a nurse, you may feel that your whole life revolves around education. You may be eager for a job that you can "leave" after eight hours. Being a nurse, however, is much more than an 8-hour job. You may have already discovered that.

Nurses cannot help but be aware of health problems that they see in their communities and daily lives. As your knowledge and experience grows, you will realize that there are innumerable concerns awaiting attention. Some may be very small things that will mean much to someone. You can arrange for someone to mend a broken porch step for an older neighbor. Maybe you can do it yourself! Some matters for consideration may require government action.

The importance of being perceptive cannot be overemphasized. You cannot be actively involved in every community health issue, but you can become knowledgeable and more aware by reading newspapers and paying attention to newscasts.

Nursing Organizations

It is important that you join a nursing organization. Perhaps you have become a member while attending school. Most nursing organizations strive to provide informational meetings and help to members. They also work for health issues in state and national legislative groups. Some organizations may function as negotiators for employee contracts and benefits. There are numerous nursing organizations, table 12–2. There are also groups who share special interests. There may be a group for nurses who are employed in home health care, or a group for clinic nurses. You may collect data about several organizations before selecting one to join.

Belonging to an organization means commitment—to attend meetings, monthly or less often, and to pay dues. Large organizations have offices and staff to maintain, so fees are needed. You may be asked to serve on a special committee, such as home health regulation. This can be very rewarding involvement; you will learn much from participating in it. The staff employees of nursing organizations include many nurses. Most organizations have regular newsletters or magazines to communicate with members.

Health-Related Organizations

Part of your community involvement may include joining a group with a special health-related interest. You have heard of groups for the mentally

Table 12–2 National nursing organizations

ORGANIZATION	MEMBERS
American Nurses Association (ANA) (State Associations are affiliated)	RNs
National Association for Practical Nurse Education and Service (NAPNES)	RNs, LP/VNs, and others interested
National Federation of Licensed Practical Nurses (NFLPN) (State groups are affiliated)	LP/VNs
National League for Nursing	RNs, LP/VNs, and others interested
National Licensed Practical Nurses' Association (NLPNA) (State groups are affiliated)	LP/VNs and students
National Student Nurses' Association (Affiliated with ANA)	Students of RN-preparing schools

handicapped, and for people with arthritis, diabetes, or strokes. Sometimes these are called *support groups*. Support groups are made up of people with similar problems. They discuss matters of concern and give each other emotional support as well as suggest ways to better cope with the problem. These groups may include the patient and/or the family.

Some groups also offer informational sessions for the public, sponsor workshops for nurses and others, and contribute to the total health scene

- Alcoholics Anonymous
- Alzheimer's Disease and Related Disorders
- American Cancer Society
    Can Surmount
    I Can Cope
    Reach to Recovery
- American Diabetes Association
- American Foundation for the Blind
- American Heart Association
- American Lung Association
- American Red Cross
- Anorexia Nervosa and Related Eating Disorders
- Arthritis Foundation
- Cystic Fibrosis Foundation
- International Agency for the Prevention of Blindness
- Medic Alert Organ Donor Program
- Mental Retardation Association of America
- Muscular Dystrophy Association
- National Hospice Organization
- National Kidney Foundation
- National Sudden Infant Death Syndrome Foundation
- United Parkinson Foundation
- United Cerebral Palsey Association

Figure 12–3 Some health-related organizations

in other ways. The Red Cross offers a variety of classes to anyone interested, from First Aid to CPR, water safety to babysitting. The American Cancer Society holds frequent workshops for nurses and also provides educational films and brochures for schools.

Nurses can join many of these groups, as a nurse or as a concerned citizen, or as a patient. It is important to recognize the concerns of patients. Sometimes nurses and other caregivers can become so involved with the problems that we forget to listen to the patient. It is important to recognize the patient's needs. Figure 12–3 lists some health-related groups.

Civic Involvement

Nurses are the largest single group of health care workers in this country. United, nurses could wield great political power. The future of health care delivery should be a concern for all nurses, whether employed or not; nurses should be involved in making such plans.

Civic involvement means power at the ballot box. In local government as well as on a broader scope, your vote is important. Also, when you are aware and concerned, the influence you have on those around you can be reflected in the ways they vote.

Active involvement in politics begins with the grass roots political organizations in your state. Some states have caucus meetings that are open to all. You should learn about health care legislation being discussed by your state legislators and on the national level. Laws that change the way health care is delivered can affect your practice and employment.

You should know about your local government and who the leaders are. Know your state legislators personally or by name. How do they feel about health related issues? What is their philosophy about quality of health care? Do they think home health care should be more strictly regulated?

KEY CONCEPT: NURSES HAVE POLITICAL POWER

- Increase your awareness of health issues.
- Belong to at least one nursing organization.
- Join other health-related groups
- Be an active citizen.

Your input about health issues is valued. Attend the city or town meetings and hearings where health issues are discussed. Write your congresspersons about your concerns. Many legislators report that form letters do not have much impact, but personal letters from constituents do receive attention. What could happen to health care if nurses would speak with one voice?

SUMMARY

Nurses are influential. Patients, families, friends, and acquaintances listen to nurses. Nurses can help promote health whether or not they are employed in nursing. While others may disagree about defining quality health care, nurses go about giving it. Care, concern, and compassion, coupled with efficiency and effort, make the bedside nurse a quality caregiver.

Nurses need to become aware of their influence and exercise it in the political world. Through participation in organizations, nurses can increase their influence to improve the future health care of people throughout the world.

FOR DISCUSSION

- Give some examples of ways in which you have informally promoted health in your neighborhood.
- How do you define quality health care? What makes people define it differently?
- Observe nurses in their daily work. What are some ways that they are contributing to quality care?
- Find out what nursing organizations are active in your area, and what they consider their primary goals. Which groups can you join? Which would you consider joining?
- Do you know how to contact your state and national legislators? If not, find out.
- What goals do you have for your life in the next 20 years? Will you be employed in health care?
- What will nursing be like in the twenty-first century?

QUESTIONS FOR REVIEW

1. List two formal and two informal ways that nurses can promote health.
2. Explain the economic philosophy of quality health care.
3. Explain the *quality-at-any-cost* philosophy of health care.
4. List three ways nurses can contribute to quality care.
5. How can nurses become more aware of health care issues?
6. Identify three national nursing organizations.

APPENDIX A

APPROVED NURSING DIAGNOSIS NORTH AMERICAN NURSING DIAGNOSIS ASSOCIATION 1986

Activity Intolerance
Activity Intolerance, Potential
Adjustment, Impaired *
Airway Clearance, Ineffective
Anxiety
Body Temperature, Potential Alteration in *
Bowel Elimination, Alteration in: Constipation
    Diarrhea
    Incontinence

Breathing Pattern, Ineffective
Cardiac Output, Alteration in: Decreased
Comfort, Alteration in: Pain
  Chronic Pain *
Communication, Impaired: Verbal
Coping, Family: Potential for Growth
Coping, Ineffective Family: Compromising
  Disabling

Coping, Ineffective Individual
Diversional Activity, Deficit
Family Process, Alteration in
Fear
Fluid Volume, Alternation In: Excess
Fluid Volume Deficit, Actual

*diagnoses accepted in 1986
Courtesy of the North American Nursing Diagnosis Association, St. Louis, MO

Fluid Volume Deficit, Potential
Gas Exchange, Impaired
Grieving, Anticipatory
Grieving, Dysfunctional
Growth and Development, Altered *
Health Maintenance, Alteration in
Home Maintenance, Management, Impaired
Hopelessness *
Hyperthermia *
Hypothermia *
Incontinence, Functional *
           Reflex *
           Stress *
           Total *
           Urge*
Infection, Potential for *

Injury, Potential for:	poisoning
	suffocation
	trauma

Knowledge Deficit (specify)
Mobility, Impaired Physical
Neglect, Unilateral*
Noncompliance (specify)

Nutrition, Alteration in:	Less than Body Requirements
	More than Body Requirements
	Potential for More than Body Requirements

Oral Mucous Membrane, Alteration in

Parenting, Alteration in:	Actual
	Potential

Post Trauma Response*
Powerlessness
Rape Syndrome

Self-Care Deficit:	feeding, bathing/hygiene
	dressing/grooming, toileting
Self Concept, Disturbance in:	body image, self-esteem, role performance, personal identity
Sensory-Perceptual Alteration:	visual, auditory, gustatory, kinesthetic, tactile olfactory

Sexual Dysfunction
Sexuality Patterns, Altered*

Skin Integrity, Impairment of:	Actual
	Potential

Sleep Pattern Disturbance
Social Interaction, Impaired*
Social Isolation
Spiritual Distress (distress of the human spirit)
Swallowing, Impaired*

APPENDIX A

Thermoregulation, Ineffective*
Thought Processes, Alteration in
Tissue Integrity, Impaired*
Tissue Perfusion, Alteration in: cerebral, cardiopulmonary
    renal, gastrointestinal, peripheral
Urinary Elimination, Alteration in Patterns
Urinary Retention*
Violence, Potential for: self-directed or directed at others

APPENDIX B

HOME HEALTH: SAMPLE ASSESSMENT AND CARE PLAN

I. DATA COLLECTION: General information
   A. Patient's initials **G D** Age *82* Date of visit *8–8*
   B. Family/home status:
      Lives with wife in townhouse. Clean, well-kept. First floor.
   C. Family/support persons:
      Wife, age 74, in pretty good health; had been caregiver until recent back injury. Neighbors, friends available.
   D. Health care professionals: Family physician (Y) N
      1. Specialists:
         Saw arthritis specialist few years ago
      2. Others: (PT, OT, etc.)
         None at present, PT taught wife how to transfer in and out of wheelchair.
      3. Reason for nurse's visit:
         Referred by doctor for home health care assessment. Patient recently hospitalized for bacterial pneumonia, and wife injured back yesterday.
   E. Major health concerns in last five years:
      Arthritis, stomach surgery for ulcer when much younger, pneumonia last week, frequent infections.
   F. Medications used: (prescribed or OTC)
      Lasix, 20 mg daily
      Digoxin, 0.25 mg daily
      Theodur, 250 mg twice daily
      Naprosyn, 375 mg twice daily
      Extra strength Tylenol, one or two every four hours as needed for pain
      Metamucil, two Tbs. at bedtime
      "Pain pills" if needed (Tylenol #3)
      Anspor, 250 mg four times daily for 10 days
   G. Current use of community services:
      Noon meals delivered from Senior Center 2 or 3 times a week

II. DATA COLLECTION: Physical health, system review
   A. Sensory
      1. Condition of skin, nails:
         Pale, thin skin. Fingernails clean and short. No bruises or skin tears noted.
      2. Vision status:
         Wears tri-focals, last exam six months ago.
      3. Hearing status:
         Watches mouths. Asks questions, words have to be repeated. Wife states some deafness is present.
      4. Known problems?
         Possible slight deafness, age-related. Has not been assessed for hearing aide.
   B. Musculoskeletal
      1. Condition of joints:
         Fingers misshapen from arthritis. Some limited motion of shoulders. All joints of lower extremities affected by arthritis. No pain at present time.
      2. Condition of muscles, tendons:
         Slight atrophy of extremities.
      3. Ambulatory status:
         Unable to walk more than few steps. Uses wheelchair between bedroom and living room. Walks from hallway into bathroom. Activity is tiring.
      4. Known problems?
         Rheumatoid arthritis past 20 years, progressively worse, not in pain now.
   C. Gastrointestinal
      1. Condition of teeth/dentures:
         Upper and lower dentures, wears during day. Appear to fit OK.
      2. Eating, digestion patterns:
         Prefers small meals, snacks. Likes many foods. Often has cheese, crackers, or chocolate as snack, small glass beer with supper.
      3. Food allergies, intolerances:
         Limits fried foods since stomach surgery.
      4. Usual diet:
         Ordinary foods, wife limits use of salt in cooking.
      5. Intestinal function:
         OK, uses Metamucil regularly
      6. Known problems?
         Occasional intolerance if upset. Pain pills cause constipation.
   D. Cardiovascular
      1. Vital Signs: T *98.2*   P *78, reg.*   R *32*   BP *156/88*
      2. Status of extremities:
         No varicosities, CMS of feet OK, some bilateral ankle edema noted.
      3. Tolerance of activity:
         Fatigues easily
      4. Known problems?
         Hypertension, probable age-related CHF (congestive heart failure).
   E. Respiratory
      1. Respiratory effort:
         Appears quite dyspneic, even when sitting. States he has productive cough when awaking.

APPENDIX B

      2. Color:
          Pale, no cyanosis. Nailbeds pale.
      3. Environmental influences:
          Quit smoking 2 years ago. Home is air-conditioned.
      4. Known problems?
          "Breathing trouble." Recovering from pneumonia. Possibly some age-related deficit.
  F. Endocrine *Not Applicable*
      1. Diabetes? Y (N)   Type I   Type II
        a. Diet:

        b. Insulin:

        c. Oral hypoglycemic:

        d. Related problems:

      2. Other known endocrine problems?
          "None"
  G. Nervous
      1. Neuro check:
          Pupils reactive, equal.
      2. Extremity function:
          Movement of upper extremities OK, lower less flexible.
      3. Speech:
          Clear, wide vocabulary.
      4. Orientation:
          Oriented to TPP (time, place, person).
      5. Known problems?
          "None"
  H. Genitourinary
      1. Bladder function:
          No problem. Up once each night.
      2. Menstrual history:
          NA
      3. Breast changes:
          NA
      4. Prostate problems:
          None
      5. Known problems?
          None

III. DATA COLLECTION: Psychosocial Health
  A. Memory
      1. Orientation to TPP:
          Oriented
      2. Past and recent events:
          No apparent memory problem

B. Thinking abilities
   1. Problem-solving:
      Clear, makes own decisions about use of pain meds
   2. Decision making:
      Speaks mind willingly
C. Communication
   1. One-to-one:
      Attentive, listens, speaks OK
   2. Groups:
      Participates in conversation, initiates topics, asks relevant questions. Asks to have some things repeated occasionally.
   3. Telephone/TV/Newspaper:
      Enjoys TV and paper. Main source of contact with outside world. Seldom uses phone, can't always hear well enough.
D. Social Network
   1. Family:
      Wife in home. Five adult children live out of town but are concerned. One is near enough to help on monthly visit.
   2. Friends/neighbors:
      Several available. One man comes every Thursday to play Yahtzee.
   3. Church/clubs:
      Was active when younger, now becomes too tired to participate. Wheelchair makes going out too hard. Minister visits every 6–8 weeks.
   4. Past and present roles:
      Managed grocery store. Was part of church committees, neighborhood groups in previous home.
   5. Community involvement:
      Follows events, cannot participate anymore.
E. Economic and financial status:
   Pension and Social Security. Medicare only. Has some savings from sale of home two years ago. Bought townhouse, put rest ($8,000) in CDs (certificates of deposit).

IV DATA COLLECTION: Environmental health
  A. Safety factors
     1. Electrical equipment:
        Home appears well kept, no hazards. Building complex was new two years ago, built to Federal guidelines for elderly housing.
     2. Appliances (walker, wheelchair, etc.):
        Wheelchair new six months ago.
     3. Pathways (floor, stairs):
        Avoids stairs. Outside steps have good rail. Some throw rugs noted on floors. Bathroom doorway too narrow for wheelchair.
     4. Furnishings:
        Adequate, comfortable. Several easy chairs and small sofa in living room. Twin beds.
  B. Space/lighting/comfort:
     Good lighting in newer construction. Wife has arranged furniture to accommodate wheelchair.

APPENDIX B

    C. Personal influences (photos, plants, crafts, etc.):
       Many personal items in home, photos on walls, souvenirs of trips displayed.

V. RATIONALE: How can this person function at home?
    A. Can the person meet own needs for hygiene, toileting, dressing, grooming?
       Wife assisted with bathing and grooming. Patient dresses self with help for socks and shoes. Wife assisted walking from hallway to toilet (3 feet) and transferring from bed to wheelchair.
    B. Can this person take own medications and perform prescribed treatments?
       Wife opens bill bottles for him.
    C. Can this person complete light housekeeping tasks that are needed?
       "Doesn't do much to help anymore." Wife does housekeeping. Son does repairs when visits.
    D. Does this person interact adequately with family, friends and the community?
       "Yes". Has lived in this building for two years but knows few neighbors. Wishes more old friends were able to visit.

VI. PROBLEM IDENTIFICATION AND INITIAL CARE PLAN
    A. Major problem areas:
       1. Physical: *Activity Intolerance, Impaired Physical Mobility, Impaired Gas Exchange, Excess Fluid Volume.*
       2. Psychosocial: *Satisfactory*
       3. Environmental: *Good*
       4. Ability to function: *Self-Care Deficit, hygiene.*
    B. Problem list, developed from major problem area:
       1. *Ambulation difficulties due to arthritis and respiratory problems.*
       2. *Severe dyspnea due to respiratory infection and age-related CHF (congestive heart failure)*
       3. *Bilateral ankle edema.*
       4. *Unable to bathe self.*
    C. Initial Care Plan

Priority Problems	Nursing/Community Intervention
1. *Impaired Gas Exchange: dyspnea*	a. *Nurse visits weekly to assess lungs, VS, meds.*
	b. *Nurse contacts doctor to obtain supplemental oxygen in home.*
	c. *Nurse assists wife in raising head of bed to 30 degrees.*
2. *Excess Fluid Volume: edema*	a. *Nurse suggests periodic use of footstool or recliner.*
	b. *Nurse assesses medication.*
	c. *Nurse reviews low salt diet with wife, checks cupboards.*
3. *Self-Care Deficit: hygiene*	a. *Home health aide visits weekly to assist with bath and shampoo*

GLOSSARY

Accountability—Being held responsible for events.
Accreditation—The process of being certified as meeting certain set standards.
Activities of Daily Living (ADLs)—Daily self help which includes personal hygiene, dressing, grooming, eating, toileting.
Acute care hospital—Hospital that specializes in the treatment of people with sudden, serious illnesses.
Advanced degree—Beyond the baccalaureate level; that is, Master of Science (MS) or Arts (MA), Doctor of Science (DSc) or Philosophy (PhD).
Advocates—People who speak or write in support of other persons or causes.
Alternative care—Health care given outside the traditional settings of hospital, nursing home, or medical office.
Ambulatory Care Center—Walk-in clinic or office; care is given on site, patient goes home.
Ambulatory Surgery Center/Surgi-center—Facility or unit where people come for surgery and return home the same day.
Ancillary workers—Health care workers who assist licensed personnel; that is, nursing assistants and assistants to therapists.
Apprenticeship—Period of time during which a student learns a craft or skill by working with a master.
Assessment interview—The first meeting between the patient and the case coordinator for the purpose of data collection.
Autonomy—Being able to function independently, make decisions for oneself.
Bio-ethical issues—Situations creating ethical conflict due to the use of technology to support or affect life; such as, organ transplants and the right to die.
Burnout—State of being exhausted, worn-out, by the stresses of one's work.
Caregiver—Concerned person, often a family member, who provides the day-to-day care that enables a frail, ill, or disabled individual to live at home. Also applies to nurses or other workers hired to give such care.
Case coordinator—Nurse or other person who plans and manages the home health care of one or more patients.
Certification—Proof that established requirements have been met.
Child Abuse Laws—Laws which forbid the neglect or abuse of dependent children by their parents or others; includes mandatory reporting of suspected abuse by professional caregivers.
Community—Any group of people with common interests or circumstances; a geographical area; any special group identified by their work, ethnic origin, living areas, or other common bond.

Community Residence/Group Home—A homelike setting for a group of people with special common needs; may be temporary or permanent; that is, homes for mentally handicapped and half-way houses for recovering alcoholics.
Compliance—Following recommended treatment.
Comprehensive—Dealing with all relevant details; health care that addresses all of the patient's needs including physical care, housing, nutrition, transportation and psychosocial support.
Consumerism—Attention to the rights of the consumer.
Consumer of health care—Any person seeking and receiving health care.
Continuing education—Classes, workshops, seminars, intended to inform; not necessarily for a degree.
Continuing education units (CEUs)—Value assigned a program according to time spent; usually, one hour is equivalent to one CEU.
Convalescent facility—A health care setting specializing in care of patients who are in the recovery phase of an illness.
Cost containment—Controlling costs through special rules and regulations.
Custodial care—Long term care; care of persons who cannot recover fully, or for whom no further treatment is intended.
Day care—Care of dependent children or adults in a special setting, given when their regular caregiver is away or employed.
Decentralized—Wide distribution of facilities.
Demographers—People who study the vital statistics of populations.
Depression, The—A period of severe economic hardship for the majority of people; 1929–1935 in the United States.
Diagnostic Related Group (DRG)—A system of classifying general medical diagnoses, used to determine amounts to be reimbursed to hospitals by government payer.
Disability—Something that restricts.
Discharge planning—Process of discussing care and making arrangements with the patient and family about future care to be given after leaving the hospital.
Discriminate—To show partiality or prejudice.
Documentation—Recordkeeping of procedures and treatments performed, also known in nursing as *charting*.
Economics—Management of the income and expenditures of a business or government.
Elective surgery—Surgical procedure which the patient may choose to have done; the patient's life is not in danger without treatment; that is, repair of non-strangulated hernia, cosmetic surgery, some orthopedic procedures.
Entrepeneur—Person who organizes and manages a business which is often a new idea and has a degree of risk.
Environmental Protection Agency (EPA)—Agency of the federal government, responsible for policing the quality of the air, land and water.
Ethical dilemmas—Problems of moral judgment which are not regulated by law; that is, abortion, euthanasia, organ transplant, use of expensive technology to preserve life of a handicapped infant.
Ethics—Standards of conduct of a given group.
Ethnic—A population group with common language, customs, characteristics and history.
Expanded health care settings—Settings for care outside of traditional hospitals and nursing homes.

GLOSSARY

Extended care—See Alternative care.
Family—Group of mutually caring individuals.
    Blended—Two adults with children of previous marriages marry each other.
    Extended—Family members live elsewhere; that is, grandparents, aunts, uncles, cousins.
    Nuclear—One or two parents and biological children.
    Nontraditional—Group-living arrangement or homosexual couple.
Federalism—Agreement that ensures states and communities a degree of self-governing, independent of direct control by national officials.
Feedback—Process of getting a response.
Fee-for-service—Billing according to the service given.
Feminists—People who believe that women should have political, economic, and social rights equal to those of men.
Folk medicine—Treatment of disease, especially involving the use of herbs and other natural substances.
Futurist—One who studies the past and present in order to predict events of the future.
Gate—Entry point to the road, or pathway into a system.
Grass roots—The basic or fundamental source of support.
Gross National Product (GNP)—Total value of a nation's annual output of goods and services.
Group practice—Three or more physicians share office space and support services.
Health care delivery system—Consists of goods and services for health care, their delivery and use, and the necessary funding.
Health care industry—All services, businesses, resources and people directly or indirectly involved with health care delivery.
Health care intervention—Actions by nurses and other caregivers to promote health, prevent or cure health problems, or to assist in maintenance or rehabilitation of chronic problems.
Health care provider—An agency, business or organization which delivers a segment of health care.
Health crisis—A time of severe trouble, a condition threatening to life or well-being.
Health Maintenance Organization (HMO)—A type of prepaid health insurance which focuses on preventing illness and maintaining wellness.
Health resources—Information sources related to health concerns, such as health care professionals, neighbors, televisions, magazines.
Health risk—Situations, events, behaviors which threaten the health of persons or communities; examples are smoking, chemical abuse, water pollution.
High-tech—Specialized technology, especially involving computerized equipment and automated machinery.
Hill-Burton Act—Federal legislation enacted in 1946, assisting small communities with financing to build hospitals.
Holistic—Viewing the person as a whole being, integrated, rather than only the sum of parts.
Homebound—Unable to go outside of one's home, usually due to physical limitation.
Home care—Taking care of the homebound person, including personal hygiene of the patient and homemaking tasks.
Home health care—Health care provided in the patient's home.

Home health care programs—Organizations providing for home health care.
   Hospital-based—Program operated from a hospital.
   Proprietary—Program operated as a private business.
   Public—Program operated as a government service.
Hospice—A philosophy of providing care for the dying patient and the family.
Hyperalimentation—Infusion of a nutrient-rich formula into a central vein.
Illness care—Care of the sick person, focusing on the cause of the illness.
Indigent—A person with limited income and no permanent address.
Inflation—Increasing costs for provided services.
Inner city—The center section of a large city, usually including a business section, and densely populated.
Intermittent skilled nursing—Care given by a licensed nurse for an hour or more on a daily or weekly basis.
Job description—Written summary of the responsibilities of a position.
Joint Commission on Accreditation of Hospitals (JCAH)—A voluntary organization which oversees hospital policies and establishes regulations to insure quality care.
Kangaroo pump—One type of electronically controlled infusion pump, often used for gastrostomy feedings.
Labor unions—An association of workers to promote and protect the welfare, interests and rights of its members, often by collective bargaining.
Latch key children—Young children who carry a key to their home and are without adult supervision from time after school until a parent or adult returns.
Liability insurance—Insurance against being held responsible for an incident causing harm.
Liaison—Connecting people or groups in order to coordinate activities; the person who is the connection.
Licensure—Granting permission to practice nursing, based on successful completion of State Board Examination.
   Inactive—In some states, a nurse who does not intend to be employed as a nurse may request placement on an inactive list.
   Mandatory—A license is required for nurse to practice for hire.
   Permissive—Licenses are granted, but not required.
Life expectancy—Statistical average of how long a person may be expected to live.
Lobby—Attempt to influence legislators regarding special interests.
Long term care facility—Health care institution providing care over a long period of time, often the remainder of the person's life.
Medicaid (Title 19, Social Security Amendments)—Provides reasonably complete medical care for the financially oppressed, regardless of age.
Medicare (Title 18, Social Security Amendments)—Government health insurance program, intended primarily for persons 65 or over.
Maintenance care—Care given only to maintain a person's life. See Custodial care.
Means test—Measure of income to determine whether a person qualifies for financial aid.
Minority population—A racial, religious, ethnic, or political group smaller than and differing from the larger, controlling group in a community, nation, etc.
Mortality—Proportion of deaths to the population of an area or nation.

GLOSSARY

National Health Care Policy—Proposals include national funding for health care for all citizens; non-existant in the United States.

Nationalism—The philosophy that national interest is more important than individual or states' rights.

Nontraditional health practices—Practices that fall outside of commonly accepted medical practice, such as folk medicine or acupuncture.

Nurse generalist—Nurse with a basic nursing education who knows about many common problems and therapies, and understands human behavior.

Nurse practitioner—Nurse who has specialized in an area of practice, often with additional education and certification; examples are pediatric practitioners, nurse midwives, and gerontological practitioners.

Nursing diagnosis—Identification of a patient's health care need based on data collection and assessment.

Occupational Safety and Health Act (OSHA)—Legislation creating government agency that oversees environmental safety in industry and workplace.

Older Americans Act—Legislation passed in 1965 creating many services for older Americans.

> **Title III**—Revision of 1982 provides for state and area Agencies on Aging (AoA) to develop comprehensive services for older persons including nutrition programs.

Ombudsman—Someone whose job is to independently investigate citizens' complaints against government agencies, serves as a liaison between the people and the government.

Outpatient—A patient treated in a clinic or emergency room and sent home.

Party—Person or organization concerned in a legal matter; the groups involved in paying for health care.

> **First party**—The patient.
> **Second party**—The health care provider.
> **Third party**—The insurance company or government program which pays for health care services.
> **Fourth party**—The employer who pays the health insurance premiums.

Personalized care—Health care designed to meet the needs of one person.

Politics—Practical wisdom, diplomacy.

Poor House—Historically, an institution for the care of those who were unable to financially support themselves; the institution was supported by public funds.

Preferred Provider Organization (PPO)—A form of HMO which allows patients to consult specialists outside of the group and pay a portion of their fees.

Prepayment—Paying for services before they are needed.

Private duty nurse—A nurse hired independently by a patient or family.

Public health nurse (PHN)—A nurse with an advanced degree, educated to care for patients in public agencies and home health care.

Public policy—A plan or course of action concerning all of the people.

Public vs. private programs—Public programs are available to all citizens and funded by taxes; private programs require private funding.

Quack—An untrained person who practices medicine or healing fraudulently; someone who pretends to have knowledge or skill.

Quality of care—A measure of the excellence of care received.

Rationale—Explanation of the reasons or basis.

Referral—Directing someone to an authority or other source.

Regulation—Rule, ordinance or law.
Reimbursement—Payment for services.
  Prospective—Payment given prior to services rendered.
  Retrospective—Payment given after services rendered.
Respite—An interval of temporary rest.
Resumé—A summary of a job applicant's experience, education and qualifications.
Screening services—Program that collects certain data about patients to determine whether or not they need further services.
Second opinion—Seeking an opinion regarding diagnosis or treatment from a second doctor.
Sheppard-Towner Act—Legislation passed in 1921 providing federal funds for nutrition, hygiene, education and equipment to aid pregnant women.
Single room occupant (SRO)—Hotels and rooming houses which rent rooms to individuals who live alone; tenants are often indigent, mentally handicapped, or chemically dependent.
Skilled care—Nursing care given by nurses and assistants.
Sliding-scale fees—Charges for services are adjusted according to the patient's ability to pay; someone with limited income will pay only a small charge.
Socialized medicine—System supplying complete medical and hospital care with public funds for all the people in the nation.
Social Security Act—Original federal legislation (1935) provided supplemental income for persons at retirement. Many amendments have occurred. See Medicare, Medicaid.
Social services—Activities designed to promote the welfare of the group and the individual; that is, counseling, health clinics, other aid for the needy, aged, or handicapped.
Standards of practice—A level of excellence considered acceptable for members of an occupation or profession.
Subsidize—Government financial support to a private business for the public good.
Subscriber—Person who contracts with an insurance company.
Support groups—People with similar concerns or problems, who meet together to discuss and share those concerns; examples are "I Can Cope," AA (Alcoholics Anonymous), Al-Anon (families of alcoholics).
Support workers—Persons who are employed in the health care industry but not directly involved in patient care; examples include clerical staff, kitchen workers, maintenance persons.
Swing beds—Beds in hospitals approved for respite services; can be adjusted for acute care patients or respite patients, depending on the need.
Target population—A group of people who are the focus of a program or who will be helped by a program.
Telephone triage—Sorting data given by patients to determine the urgency of medical attention.
Volunteer agencies—A service group manned predominately by unpaid workers; the Red Cross is a well-known example.
Vulnerable adult—An adult who is physically or financially dependent on others.
Watch dog(s)—Person or group that observes government functions in order to prevent waste, fraud, or unethical practices.

BIBLIOGRAPHY

ARTICLES

"American health care: a system in crisis," *Healthline*. vol. 2, no. 10. The Robert A. McNeil Foundation for Health Education (October 1983): 7–9.

Barthkowski, J. and Swandby, J. "Charting nursing's course through megatrends." *Nursing and Health Care*, vol. 6, no. 9. (September 1985): 375.

Behrens, E. "Charting your success with an effective resume." *LPN*. (Spring 1986): 14–18.

Bernzweig, E. "Avoiding the legal pitfalls of home care," *RN*. (August 1986): 49–50.

Boyle, J. "The challenges of health care in America," *Vital Speeches of the Day*. Southold, NY: City News Publishing Co. (May 1, 1985): 426–429.

Butrin, J. "Day care: a new idea?" *Journal of Gerontological Nursing*. vol. 11, no. 4. (April, 1985): 19–22.

Califano, J. "A revolution looms in American health," *The New York Times*, March 25, 1986.

"The corporate Rx for Medical Costs," *Business Week*. (Oct. 15, 1984): 138–139.

DeYoung, H. G. "Health care looks beyond the Hospital." *High Technology*. (Sept., 1985); 46–51.

Dirschel, K. "A mandate for standards of care," *Nursing and Health Care*, vol. 7, no. 1. (January 1986): 27–29.

Dunn, J. "Warning: giving telephone advice is hazardous to your professional health," *Nursing 85*. vol. 15, no. 8. (August 1985): 40–41.

Edler, C. "If a friend asks you for medical advice," *RN*. (August 1986): 38–40.

Edwardson, S. "Shedding light on a shifting marketplace: competition in maternity care," *Nursing and Health Care*, vol. 7, no. 2. (February 1986): 73–77.

Fair, J. "Reflections on images," *LPN*. (Fall 1985): 4, 29.

Felton, G. "Harnassing today's trends to guide nursing's future," *Nursing and Health Care*, vol. 7, no. 4. (April 1986): 211–213.

Francis, B. "Nursing care: a cultural approach," *LPN*. (Winter, 1986): 6–9, 19.

Friedman, J. "Guiding patients through the labyrinth of home health care services," *Nursing and Health Care*, vol. 7, no. 6. (June 1986): 305–306.

Griffin, Sr. S., Peterson, Sr. D., and Brower, H. T. "The problems and payoffs of setting up a rural health clinic," *Nursing and Health Care,* vol. 7, no. 2. (February 1986): 79–82.

Griffith, D. "Blending key ingredients to assure quality home care," *Nursing and Health Care.* vol. 7, no. 6. (June 1986): 301–302.

Griffith, H. "Who will become the preferred providers?" *American Journal of Nursing.* vol. 85, no. 5. (May 1985): 538–542.

Hall, B. and Allan, J. "Sharpening nursing's focus by focusing on health," *Nursing and Health Care* vol. 7, no. 6. (June 1986): 315–320.

Hanley, R. "Cost containment of health care," *Vital Speeches.* (Nov. 15, 1984): 74–77.

"Health insurers are cracking down on scams," *Business Week.* (October 15, 1984): 140–143.

Horner, D. "The battle for control of health care," *Vital Speeches.* (Nov. 15, 1984): 93–96.

Jackson, A. "High tech's influence on our lives," *Vital Speeches.* (Jan. 1, 1985): 164–166.

Joel, L. "DRGs: the state of the art of reimbursement for nursing services," *Nursing and Health Care,* vol. 4, no. 12. (December 1983): 560–563.

Johns, J. "Self-care today–in search of an identity," *Nursing and Health Care,* vol. 6, no. 3. (March 1985): 153–156.

Kuhn, M. "Nurses and patients—together we can heal the sick health care system." *Nursing and Health Care.* vol. 6, no. 7. (September 1985): 363–364.

Lamm, R. "Anti-social ethics: health care costs," *Vital Speeches.* (Mar. 15, 1985): 325–327.

Lauver, E. "Where will the money go? Economic forecasting and nursing's future." *Nursing and Health Care.* vol. 6, no. 3. (March 1985): 133–135.

"The life-and-death choices created by medical technology." *Business Week.* (Oct. 15, 1984): 144–146.

McHatton, M. "A theory for timely teaching," *American Journal of Nursing,* vol. 85, no. 7. (July 1985): 798–800.

Messner, R. and Darby, L. "Hospice: a new horizon for nurses," *The Journal of Practical Nursing.* (September 1985): 30–31.

Miller, A. "When is the time ripe for teaching?" *American Journal of Nursing.* vol. 85, no. 7. (July 1985): 801–804.

Minnesota Department of Labor and Industry. "Employee right-to-know Act of 1983." State of Minnesota, 1985.

National Advisory Council on Vocational Education. "The education of nurses: a rising national concern—position paper." *Issue Paper No. 2.* May 1980.

O'Leary, J. "What employers will expect from tomorrow's nurses," *Nursing and Health Care,* vol. 7, no. 4. (April 1986): 207–209.

Patricelli, R. "Health care reform." *Vital Speeches.* (Nov. 1, 1984): 38–42.

Shaffer, F. "DRGs: history and overview," *Nursing and Health Care.* vol. 4, no. 9. (September 1983): 388–396.

Smith, C. "DRGs: making them work for you." *Nursing 85.* vol. 15, no. 1. (January 1985): 34–41.

"Special day care" Nurse's Notebook. *Nursing 86.* vol. 16, no. 3. (March 1986): 87.

Stone, M. "Rampaging health costs," *U.S. News and World Report.* (Mar. 26, 1984): 84.

"Tender loving care Inc." *TIME.* (Feb. 17, 1986): 57.

"Ten trends to watch," *Nursing and Health Care,* vol. 7, no. 1. (January 1986): 17–19.

Thobaben, M. and Anderson, L. "Reporting elder abuse: it's the law," *American Journal of Nursing.* vol. 85, no. 4. (April 1985): 371–374.

Toufexis, A. "Just tick, tick, ticking along," *TIME.* (Dec. 17, 1984): 79.

U.S. Bureau of the Census. *Statistical Abstract of the United States: 1986* (106th Ed) Washington, 1985.

Wajdowicz, E. "The americanization of Florence: a look at associate degree nurses," *Nursing and Health Care.* vol. 7, no. 2. (February 1986): 97–99.

Wakefield–Fisher, M., Wright, M., and Kraft, L. "A First for the Nation: North Dakota and Entry into Nursing Practice." *Nursing and Health Care,* vol. 7, no. 3. (March 1986): 135–141.

Walker, L. "Nursing diagnoses and interventions: new tools to define nursing's unique role," *Nursing and Health Care.* vol. 7, no. 6. (June 1986): 323–326.

Wallis, C. "Another setback in Louisville," *TIME* (May 6, 1985): 64.

Ward, D. "Why patient teaching fails fails fails," *RN.* (January 1986): 45–47.

Waters, S. "What it's really like to work in an ambulatory care center." *RN* (May 1985): 51–53.

Waters, S. "What happens if your hospital bills separately for nursing?" *RN.* (July 1985): 18–21.

BOOKS

Baxandall, R., Gordon, L., and Reverby, S., Ed. *America's Working Women: A Documentary History—1600 to the Present.* New York: Random House Inc., 1976.

Becker, B. and Fendler, D. *Vocational and Personal Adjustments in Practical Nursing.* 5th ed. St. Louis: The C. V. Mosby Co., 1986.

Bullough, B., Bullough, V., and Soukap, M. *Nursing Issues and Nursing Strategies for the Eighties.* New York: Springer Publishing Co., 1983.

Burgess, W., and Ragland, E. *Community Health Nursing Philosophy, Process, Practice.* Norwalk, CT: Appleton–Century–Crofts, 1983.

Carpenito, L. *Handbook of Nursing Diagnosis.* Philadelphia: J. B. Lippincott Co., 1984.

Community Health Nursing: Education and Practice. New York: NLN, 1980.

Corr, C. and Corr, D., eds. *Hospice Care Principles and Practice.* New York: Springer Publishing Co., 1983.

Dahl, R. *Democracy in the United States: Promise and Performance,* 4th ed. Boston: Houghton Mifflin Co., 1981.

Diseases, Nurses' Reference Library. Nursing 84 Books, Springhouse, PA: Springhouse Publishing, 1984.

Doenges, M., Jeffries, M., and Moorhouse, M. *Nursing Care Plans, Nursing Diagnoses in Planning Patient Care.* Philadelphia: F. A. Davis Co, 1984.

Eisenberg, D. *Encounters with Gi: Exploring Chinese Medicine.* New York: W. W. Norton Co. Inc., 1985.

Ellis, J. and Nowlis, E. *Nursing: A Human Needs Approach.* Boston: Houghton Mifflin Co., 1985.

Falkson, J. *HMOs and the Policies of Health System Reform.* Chicago: American Hospital Association, 1980.

Frommer, M. *Community Health Care and the Nursing Process,* 2nd ed. St. Louis: The C. V. Mosby Co., 1983.

Holman, A. *Family Assessment: Tools for Understanding and Intervention.* Beverly Hills, Sage Publications, 1983.

Hutchison, M. *Megabrain: New Tools and Techniques for Brain Growth and Mind Expansion.* New York: William Morrow & Co., 1986.

Lesner, P. *Pediatric Nursing.* Albany, NY: Delmar Publishers Inc., 1983.

Mayer, T. and Mayer, G. *The Health Insurance Alternative.* New York: Putman Publishing, 1984.

McAdoo, H., Ed. *Black Families.* Beverly Hills, Sage Publications, 1981.

Milliken, M. *Understanding Human Behavior,* 3rd Ed. Albany, NY: Delmar Publishers Inc., 1981.

Milliken, M., and Campbell, G. *Essential Competencies for Patient Care.* St. Louis: The C. V. Mosby Co., 1985.

Nassif, J. *The Home Health Care Solution.* New York: Harper & Row, 1985.

Olson, David H. et al. *Families—What Makes them Work.* Beverly Hills, Sage Publications, 1983.

Panos, M. and Heimlich, J. *Homeopathic Medicine at Home.* Los Angeles: J. P. Tarcher, Inc., 1980.

Petrowski, D. *Handbook of Community Health Nursing.* New York: Springer Publishing Co., 1984.

Practices. Nurse's Reference Library, Nursing 84 Books. Springhouse, PA: Springhouse Corporation, 1984.

Scherman, S. *Community Health Nursing Care Plans: A Guide for Home Health Care Professionals.* New York: John Wiley and Sons Inc., 1985.

Spiegel, A. *Home Healthcare.* Owing Mills, MD: National Health Publishing, 1983.

Steinberg, R., and Carter, G. *Case Management and the Elderly.* Lexington, MA: Lexington Books, 1983.

Tobin, S., Davidson, S. and Sack, A. *Effective Social Services for Older Americans.* Institute of Gerontology, Univ. of Michigan—Wayne State Univ., 1976.

Townsend, C. *Nutrition and Diet Therapy,* 4th Ed. Albany, NY: Delmar Publishers Inc., 1985.

Weil, A. *Health and Healing.* Boston: Houghton Mifflin Co., 1983.

INDEX

Acupuncture, 119
Adult,
   day care, 180
   elderly adults, abuse of, 128–29, 130–31
Ambulatory care centers, 54, 56
Ambulatory surgery centers, 56
   working in, 169–74
American Hospital Association, 15
American Red Cross. *See* Red Cross
Ancillary workers, 21
Asbestosis, 82
Asian Americans, 123
Asian communities, health concerns of, 82
Assessment,
   guidelines through life span, 145–50
   nursing process and, 137–38

Barton, Clara, 20
Bio-ethical issues, 199
Biofeedback, 119
Black Americans, 123
   health concerns of, 82
Black Lung Disease, 82
Board on Aging, 40
Brown, Esther Lucile, 21
Burnout, warnings of, 187

Care planning, home health care and, 72–73
Case,
   assignment, home health care, 73–74
   conferences, home health care, 74
   coordinators, 10
Cast care, instructions for home, 166
Child abuse, 127–28
Children, day care for ill, 56–57
Children's Bureau, 30
Chiropractic, 120
Christman, Luther, 21
Civil Rights Act of 1964, 87

Clergy, home health care and, 113
Clinics, working in, 163–69
COA. *See* Council on Accreditation of Services for Families and Children
Communication,
   therapeutic, 144, 151
      guidelines for, 152
Communities,
   defined, 79
   ethnic, 81–82
   health care teams and, 95–99
      interaction between, 97
   health risk identification and resolution, 89
   involvement in health care concerns, 84–89
   nurses and, 91–92
   school, 82–84
   work related, 82
Community Action Program, 88
Community home, 57–58
Congregate dining, 85
Continuing education, 197–98
Convalescent care facilities, 57
Cost,
   containment of in health care, 41–44
      effects of, 44–48
Council on Accreditation of Services for Families and Children (COA), 71
Culture,
   health care and, 117–24
   identifying differences in, 151
Curative intervention in health care, 27–28

Day care,
   disabled or elderly adults, 58
   ill children and, 56–57
Diagnostic Related Groups (DRGs), 42–43
   costs compared with other methods, 45
Dietitians, home health care and, 114
Dix, Dorothea, 20

Doctors,
    changing roles of, 8
    home health care and, 110–11
DRGs. *See* Diagnostic Related Groups

Economic Opportunity Act, 88
Education,
    patient, 151–58
    promoting, 102–4
Elderly adult abuse, 128–29, 130–31
Emergency Maternity and Infant Care Act, 30–31
Employee Right to Know Act, 85
English poor laws, 14
Environmental Protection Agency, 25
EOA. *See* Equal Opportunity Act
Equal Opportunity Act (EOA), 30, 31
Erikson, Erik, 142
Ethnic communities, 81–82
Evaluation in the nursing process, 139–40

Fair Packaging and Labeling Act, 88
Faith healing, 120
Families
    abuse in, 127–32
        child, 127–28
        elderly adult, 128–29, 130–31
        substance, 129, 132
    acute problems of, 126
    home health care and, 110
    identifying differences in, 151
    influence on health care, 124–33
    structure of, 125–26
Federal Occupation Safety and Health Act (OSHA), 82
Fee-for-service, 35, 38–39
    compared with other payment methods, 45
Food Stamp Program, 88

Granite Cutters Union, 36

Hall, Lydia, 20
Health care,
    caregivers changing roles in, 8–9
    concerns, community involvement in, 84–89
    cost containment of, 41–44
        comparison of payment methods, 45
        effects of, 44–48

cultural influences on, 117–24
decentralization of, 4
delivery system, 12–33
    defined, 13
    history of, 14–23, 25
    public policy and, 29–32
family influences on, 124–33
federal government and, 4
future of, 3–11
    caregivers and, 3–8
    patient care and, 9–10
home. *See* Home health care
industrial growth of, 7
inflation costs chart, 42
influencing future, 202–16
intervention levels of, 23–29
    curative intervention, 27–28
    health promotion, 25–27
    maintenance and rehabilitation, 28–29
    primary prevention, 27
issues of quality in, 206–11
payment for, 35–49
    alternatives of, 35–38
    combination plans, 40
    fee-for-service, 38–39
    prepayment, 35, 39
problems, 31–32
settings for, 50–60
    ambulatory care centers, 54, 56
    ambulatory surgery centers, 56
    community homes, 57–58
    convalescent care facilities, 57
    day care for elderly or disabled adults, 58
    day care for ill children, 56–57
    factors influencing choice of, 61
    hospices, 58–60
    hospitals, 51–52
    long term care and, 53
    medical clinics, 54
    respite care, 52–53
Health care teams,
    defining, 95–99
        hospital, 96
    developing comprehensive, 99–100
    implementing successful, 100–101
    interaction with the community, 97
    nurses and, 104–5

INDEX

Health care teams (*Continued*)
  successful, 101–4
    promoting education, 102–4
    promoting wellness, 102
Health concerns,
  United States, 80–81
  world, 79–80
Health Maintenance Organizations, 8, 39
  costs compared with other methods, 45
Health promotion, 25–27, 203–5
Health-related organizations, 212–14
Health risks, identification and resolution of, 89
Henderson, Virginia, 21
Hierarchy of needs, 142
Hill–Burton Act, 21–22
Hispanic Americans, 123–24
  health concerns of, 82
HMO. *See* Health Maintenance Organizations
Home care records, 177–79
Home health care, 60, 64–75
  administration of agencies, 71–75
    care planning, 72–73
    case assignment, 73–74
    case conferences, 74
  clergy and, 113
  community and, 113
  cultural influences on, 117–24
  defined, 67
  dietitians and, 114
  doctors and, 110–11
  example of, 116–17
  family and, 110
  history of, 65–69
  home care records, 177–79
  home visitation, 176
  homemakers and, 112–13
  nurses and, 111
  patients and, 109–10
  pharmacists and, 114
  philosophy of, 68–69
  recordkeeping, 74
  regulation of agencies, 70–71
  social workers and, 115
  teachers and, 114
  terminating, 74
  therapists and, 115
  types of, 69–71

  volunteers and, 113
  working in, 174–180
Homemakers, home health care and, 112–13
Homeopathy, 120
Hospices, 58–60
  working in, 181–82
Hospitals,
  health care and, 51–52
  home health care based programs, 70
Hypnosis, 120

Implementation in the nursing process, 139
Insurance, 36
  liability, 195–96
Intervention in health care, 23–29
  curative intervention, 27–28
  health promotion, 25–27
  maintenance and rehabilitation, 28–29
  primary prevention, 27
Interviews in job seeking, 188, 191

JCAH. *See* Joint Commission on Accreditation of Hospitals
Job seeking, 188–97
  interviews, 188, 191
  resumés, 188
    examples of, 189–91
  steps in, 188
Johnson, Lyndon, 87
Joint Commission on Accreditation for Hospitals (JCAH), 22, 70

Kenny, Elizabeth, 20

Labor unions and, 196
Latch Key children, 82
Liability insurance, 195–96
Lister, Joseph, 15
Long term care, 53

Maass, Clara, 20
Mahoney, Mary Eliza, 20
Maintenance and rehabilitation in health care, 28–29
M.A.S.H., 22
Maslow, Abraham, 141
  hierarchy of needs, 142

Maternal and Child Health Care Act, 30
Medicaid, 37, 88
    home health care and, 70
    means test, 38
Medical clinics, 54
Medicare, 37–38, 88
    home health care and, 70
    Prospective Payment Plan (PPP), 42
Migraine headaches, biofeedback and, 119
Minneapolis Girls Vocational High School, 17
Montag, Mildred, 21

National health care problems, 31–32
National HomeCaring Council (NHC), 70
National Institute of Child Health and Human Development, 31
National League for Nursing (NLN), 70
National Ombudsman Association, 40
Native Americans, 122–23
Needs,
    adapting care to, 143–44
    hierarchy of, 142
NHC. See National HomeCaring Council
Nightingale, Florence, 15
NLN. See National League for Nursing
Nontraditional health practices, 118–20
Nurses,
    adapting care to needs of patients, 143–44
    burnout, warnings of, 187
    changing roles of, 8–9
    community and, 91–92
    continuing education, 197–98
    duties in 1887, 19
    ethical issues and, 197–200
    ethics of, 197
    future health care and, 202–16
    generalists, 8
    health promotion and, 203–5
    home health care and, 111
    labor unions, 196
    liability insurance and, 195–96
    political involvement and, 211–15
    responsibilities to self and career, 185–201
        job seeking, 188–97
        understanding self, 185–87
    special clinical, 8

Nursing,
    education, history of, 24
    ethical issues for, 197–200
    future of, 3–11
    home health care and, 111
    technical versus professional, 199–200
Nursing homes, 53
Nursing organizations, 212
Nursing process, 136–41
    assessment, 137–38
        guidelines through life span, 145–50
    implementation of, 139
    patient's needs and, 141–42
    planning, 138–39
    traditional and expanded contrasted, 140–41
Nutting, Mary Adelaide, 20

Older Americans Act, 27, 85
Ombudsman concept, 40
OSHA. See Federal Occupation Safety and Health Act
Outpatients,
    postoperative instructions, 155
    preoperative instructions, 154

Patients,
    adapting care to needs of, 143–44
    care, future of, 9–11
    education of, 151–58
    home health care and, 109–10
    postoperative instructions, 155
    preoperative instructions, 154
    sample situation, 159–60
Pharmacists, home health care and, 114
Physicians. See Doctors
Planning in the nursing process, 138–39
PMS. See Premenstrual syndrome
Political involvement, 211–15
Poor houses, 15
Poor laws, 14
Population, predicted changes in, 7
Postoperative instructions, 155
PPO. See Preferred Provider Organizations
PPP. See Medicare, Prospective Payment Plan
Preferred Provider Organizations (PPO), 40
Premenstrual syndrome (PMS), biofeedback and, 119

INDEX

Preoperative instructions, 154
Prepayment for service, 35, 39
Primary prevention in health care, 27
Problem solving, steps in, 198
Professional Standard Review Organizations (PSRO), 41
Project Lifesaver, 104
Proprietary agencies,
 defined, 69
 home health care and, 69–70
Prospective Payment Plan, 42
PSRO. *See* Professional Standard Review Organizations
Public health agencies, home health care and, 69
Public health nurses, 69

Quacks, defined, 119
Quality Care, Inc., 69

Recordkeeping, home health care, 74
Red Cross, 27
Respite care, 52–53
 working in, 181
Resumés, 188
 examples of, 189–91
Richards, Linda, 20
Robb, Isabel Hampton, 20
Rubin, Reva, 21

School communities, 82–84
Semmelweis, Ignaz Filipp, 15
Sheppard–Towner Act, 30
Signing, defined, 121
Social Security Act, 18, 88
 Amendments of 1963, 1965, 31
 Professional Standard Review Organizations, 41
 Title V, 30
 Title 18, 89
 Title 19, 89
Social workers, home health care and, 115
Substance abuse, 129, 132

Target population, defined, 84
Teachers, home health care and, 114
Telephone etiquette, 167
Theory of Basic Needs, 141
Therapeutic communication, 144, 151
 guidelines for, 152
Therapists, home health care and, 115
Torrop, Hilda, 21

Upjohn Health Care Service, Inc., 69

VISTA, 88
Vocational Education Act of 1948, 22
Volunteers in Service to America. *See* VISTA

Wald, Lillian D., 20
Watch dogs, defined, 78
Water Quality Act, 88
Wellness, promoting individual, 102
Wholesale Meat Act, 88
WIC. *See* Women, Infants and Children Program
Women, Infants and Children Program (WIC), 27
Women's movement, 198–99
Work Experience Program, 88
Work related communities, 82
Work settings,
 adult day care, 180
 ambulatory surgery center, 169–74
 clinics, 163–69
 home health care, 174–80
 hospice, 181–82
 respite care, 181